*Transforming the Quality of Life
for People with Dementia through
Contact with the Natural World*

Oı

by the same authors

Past Trauma in Late Life
European Perspectives on Therapeutic Work with Older People
Linda Hunt, Mary Marshall and Cherry Rowlings
ISBN 978 1 85302 446 7

Perspectives on Rehabilitation and Dementia
Edited by Mary Marshall
ISBN 978 1 84310 286 1

Dementia
New Skills for Social Workers
Edited by Alan Chapman and Mary Marshall
ISBN 978 1 85302 142 8

of related interest

Design for Nature in Dementia Care
Garuth Chalfont
ISBN 978 1 84310 571 8
Bradford Dementia Group Good Practice Guides

Transforming the Quality of Life for People with

DEMENTIA

through Contact with the

NATURAL
WORLD

Fresh Air on My Face

Edited by Jane Gilliard and Mary Marshall

Jessica Kingsley *Publishers*
London and Philadelphia

Extract from 'Wild Oats' by Norman MacCaig on p.16 is
printed with permission from Birlinn publishers.

First published in 2012
by Jessica Kingsley Publishers
116 Pentonville Road
London N1 9JB, UK
and
400 Market Street, Suite 400
Philadelphia, PA 19106, USA

www.jkp.com

Library of Congress Cataloging in Publication Data
A CIP catalog record for this book is available from the Library of Congress

British Library Cataloguing in Publication Data
A CIP catalogue record for this book is available from the British Library

ISBN 978 1 84905 267 2
eISBN 978 0 85700 544 1

Printed and bound in Great Britain

This book is dedicated to all the people with dementia currently living in long-term care who never go outside. Their plight motivated us to produce this book.

In memory of

Malcolm Goldsmith,

10 February 1939–28 July 2011,
whose wisdom helped so many people to better
understand and serve people with dementia.

Contents

Acknowledgements

We want to thank our authors, photographers and people in the photographs most warmly for their contributions. We also want to thank Jessica Kingsley, who trusted us to produce the book right from the start, and Ron Smith, who did our proof reading. We hope they all feel proud of the result and its potential to inspire more effort to connect people with dementia with nature.

Introduction

JANE GILLIARD AND MARY MARSHALL

What do we mean by nature?

How do you describe the shiver of delight you experience on hearing a blackbird sing from the top of a tree in the winter dusk? Or the sense of wonder when you see a sunset across the sea? Or the sweet softness of the velvet of a dog's ears? Or the luscious pleasure of eating a handful of freshly picked blackberries? Or the sharp, almost tear-jerking memories that overwhelm you when you smell a bonfire? Or the intense amusement of walking through autumn leaves? And of course, less positively, your anxiety at the roar of the wind, or feeling bitterly cold or soaking wet in the rain. How can we share our views that these experiences are life affirming – indeed, essential to a feeling of being alive and having a place in the grand scheme of things?

It seems that, in our secular society, talking about sensory and emotional experiences of nature is left to poets or religious people. Indeed, for some people God and nature are the same thing. The rest of us are almost embarrassed to write about them or to share how important they are. It sometimes feels as if those who talk or write about religion have bagged the language of nature for themselves.

This leads us to hesitate to talk and write about the importance for both of us of being outside, just to get through our daily lives. We walk when we need to think. We go out to clear our heads or to diminish feelings of frustration or irritation. We are calmed by being in woods, surrounded by trees far older than we are. Our lives are hugely enhanced by a walk along a beach, with the waves lapping on the sand in the sun or crashing onto the shore in a wind. We are both keen on natural history, especially watching birds and studying flowers, and we cannot imagine a life when we are not outside in the quiet, just watching wild birds or enjoying the flora.

It seems in some way ludicrous to produce a book on nature and dementia when we mammals are part of nature. We all live in the natural world with the sky above us and the earth below. Rain falls on all of us and the sun warms us. We are all accustomed to seeing trees, even in the busiest cities, where there are always plane trees and cherry trees. People with dementia are in the same world, so why do we feel there is a need for this book? The answer is that we are concerned that people with dementia are often not able to experience the natural world. They often live inside all the time. About a third of people with dementia live in care homes (National Audit Office 2007). They live in artificial light most of the time. Their window constrictors limit the amount of fresh air they can breathe. We know from the SCRC/MWC (Scottish Commission for the Regulation of Care/Mental Welfare Commission) research that 50 per cent of people with dementia in care homes never go out of the home, and another 25 per cent go out rarely (Care Commission and Mental Welfare Commission 2009). This may mean that they go into the gardens – but the authors comment on the under-use of gardens, even if they are specially designed for people with dementia. Even people with dementia who live at home can lose their confidence about going outside, or may live with anxious relatives who discourage it. This is in sharp contrast with prisoners, who are required to be allowed an hour outside each day.[1]

Not being able to go outside is a possible future that chills us. We feel equally concerned that even if we were allowed in the garden, it would be only when the weather was ideal, and we would never have an opportunity to feel the wind or rain on our faces, or crunch the snow beneath our feet. Furthermore, we would never be allowed to go outside the garden into the wilder places we love. Being outside provides a rich combination of multi-sensory stimulation and emotion. Who could not feel, either when rain runs down their face or they smell the soil as rain begins to fall?

We see children full of wonder at the natural world, and it may be that as you get older it becomes easier to reconnect with this. It seems to us incontrovertible that nature becomes more important as you get older, and this may be even more true when cognition is impaired and feelings and emotions are even stronger. Peter Whitehouse and his colleagues describe a project which links children and people with dementia in learning about and appreciating nature.

---

1   Prison Rules 1999, section 30: 'If the weather permits and subject to the need to maintain good order and discipline, a prisoner shall be given the opportunity to spend time in the open air at least once every day, for such a period as may be reasonable in the circumstances.'

Many people, such as farmers and fishermen, have had a lifetime outside. For others their activities outside are their consuming passion – for example, sailors, riders, walkers and birders. For these people their sense of self is profoundly related to the outside world. But then all of us spend a lot of time outside, even just doing everyday things like waiting for a bus or walking in the park, and for us too, our complete selves will include the experience of being outside. We would assert that people must remain in touch with nature to be whole beings. John Zeisel (2011) says we are all hard-wired to need contact with nature, which is one way of putting it for inhibited twenty-first-century people in dementia care.

It is possible to talk about this need for nature in instrumental terms. We all need fresh air, sunlight, exercise, and to breathe properly, for our health. Many outside activities are social and enhance our social selves. These reasons are really important and are a lot easier to talk about than the sensory and emotional importance of being outside. Perhaps we need to emphasise the pragmatic reasons for being outside if we are to convince professionals of the importance of it. Notably, Enhancing the Healing Environment (EHE) projects for improving the environment of acute general hospitals for people with dementia often include bringing nature into the wards.[2]

Dementia

So far we have shared our concerns that people with dementia might not have the contacts with nature that they want and need, but we pause for a moment to brief the readers who do not have a background in dementia care. 'Dementia' is an umbrella term for a group of progressive diseases of the brain, including Alzheimer's disease, vascular dementia and Lewy body dementia. In our view, people with alcohol-related brain damage (ARDB) share a great many experiences and needs with people with dementia (although their condition is not, strictly speaking, progressive). The common impairments of dementia include impaired memory (especially recent memory), impaired reasoning and learning impairment. Most people with dementia are older people, so they will also have impairments associated with ageing, and typically of eyesight and hearing, which are particularly problematic because the dementia will prevent them understanding and dealing with them. There are

---

2   See www.enhancingthehealingenvironment.org.uk.

numerous other impairments but each person's pathway through the illness is different, so we resist generalising.

About 3 per cent of people with dementia are younger than 65 and have particular difficulties such as employment, and children to support. There are rapidly increasing numbers of people with dementia because it is very much associated with age and we have an ageing population. At age 65 about one in 20 people has dementia, at age 85 it is one in three or four. Ensuring expertise and experience is shared is an urgent priority. In this book we have tried to provide ideas for making contact with nature for people with all levels of impairment, although some of the activities such as walking the hills are clearly for people who are physically fitter.

This book

This book aims to wake people up to the reality that even the best care sometimes excludes contact with nature which we, and our contributors, feel is an innate need for all of us. We hope to provide some examples of ways people with dementia can enjoy nature, which will inspire and encourage people with dementia, their relatives and everyone else with an interest.

This is an opportunistic collection of interesting ideas and work rather than a themed presentation. Our aim in choosing our contributors was to find people who had not written before or had not written about this topic, including people with dementia. We contacted people with dementia whom we knew. James McKillop, Brian and June Hennell and Trevor Jarvis were willing to contribute, along with members of the excellent Scottish Dementia Working Group and the Swindon Forget Me Not Centre. We were also grateful that Hawker Publications agreed to let us use two poems by John Killick from his *Dementia Diary* collection (Killick 2009). Many of our contributors, especially Rachael Litherland and the members of the Park Club, have quoted people with dementia. Manjit Nijjar presents the views and voices of Asian carers.

We found our other contributors by talking to a lot of people, following up on people we had heard of or read about, and contacting some people we heard speak at conferences. Our contributors have very different backgrounds and approaches to their chapters, which was deliberate on our part because we felt it would provide a rich collection that would stimulate lateral thinking and imagination. We know there are significant gaps. We tried hard but failed to find people to write about wild birds, trees, quiet places, stars, the seaside, and swimming (although we are certain there is good work going on). There must be many more aspects of nature where there are interesting projects, but we were limited by our networks, time, and the size of the book. We know there is a lot of work about gardens, horticulture and plants generally and we have limited ourselves to one chapter, mainly by people with dementia, because there are many books and articles about gardens.

We start by looking at practical arguments for going outside more. There are good physical health reasons; David McNair looks at vitamin D, and the Swindon Hiking Group benefit from the exercise. There are also reasons for going outside related to coping better with intellectual impairment and many of our authors emphasise this. Two examples here: being outside can be orientating to the seasons, as Neil Mapes emphasises, and David McNair talks about improving circadian rhythm.

On a more philosophical level, Malcolm Goldsmith suggests that the need for nature is innate in all of us. Peter Whitehouse and his colleagues help us to see that we need to rethink our attitudes to dementia and to nature, and to align these more with modern thinking about sustainability. All the chapters talk about the fundamental need to relate to nature even when they are describing a particular project.

The varied professional backgrounds of our contributors have given rise to an eclectic approach to the topic. Most of them emphasise the potential of linking with nature for activities which are so crucial to the well-being of people with dementia, whose lives are often characterised by profound and disabling boredom. Marcus Fellows and Ann Rainsford, for example, emphasise the potential of animals for activities for their residents with dementia, and Lorraine Robertson likewise about tending the allotment. We are surprised that the 'farming for health' movement does not seem to have reached the UK yet to any extent. De Bruin and colleagues offer a useful description of the concept of 'farming for health' and what it can mean for people with dementia.

Our contributors have very different backgrounds and approach the topic very differently. Claire Craig, for example, who writes about creative activities, is a lecturer in occupational therapy. Halldóra Arnardóttir is an art historian and her husband and colleague Javier Sánchez Merina is an architect. Their contribution is about designing a building incorporating nature. People with dementia also talk about their enjoyment of gardens, and from Peter Whitehouse we learn about Arne Naess, who had a very profound connection with nature and who also had dementia.

Finally, we acknowledge that we have omitted one of the most important reasons for providing proximity of nature for people with dementia, which is that it provides something to watch and this can be something amusing. Perhaps we have not included enough about the entertainment value of a contact with nature. We finish this introductory chapter with a snippet from Norman MacCaig to make the point about the enjoyment of watching:

> Every day I see from my window
> pigeons, up on a roof ledge – the males
> are wobbling gyroscopes of lust.

> *Norman MacCaig,* 'Wild Oats'

Language
Our role as editors has been a real pleasure. We have made only two changes to our contributions in relation to language: we have changed all mention of 'persons' to 'people' and we have used the term 'people with dementia', which we believe is the least stigmatising.

References

Care Commission and Mental Welfare Commission (2009) *Remember I'm Still Me.* Edinburgh: Mental Welfare Commission.

Killick, J. (2009) *Dementia Diary: Poems and Prose.* London: Hawker.

McCaig, E. (2005) 'Wild Oats.' *The Poems of Norman MacCaig.* Edinburgh: Polygon.

National Audit Office (2007) *Improving Services and Support for People with Dementia.* NAO: London.

Zeisel, J. (2011) *I'm Still Here. A Breakthrough Approach to Understanding Someone Living with Alzheimer's.* London: Piatkus.

Chapter 1

Dementia, Spirituality and Nature

MALCOLM GOLDSMITH

More than a decade ago David Jenkins, the then Bishop of Durham, summing up a conference on 'Spirituality and Ageing', talked of 'spirituality' as a 'weasel of a word', complaining that it meant anything that the speaker or writer wanted it to mean, almost to the point of becoming meaningless. Since then I must have on file over 50 definitions of the word as people have grappled to describe something real in their experience which seems to defy description. This is not really a help when in discussion with others! The definition which I prefer most, because of its breadth of understanding, its attempt to make concrete abstract notions, and which is honest about its own fragility is one by the American Mel Kimble (2001), who used to work with Viktor Frankl.[1] He writes: 'The spiritual dimension is the energy within that strives for meaning and purpose, it is the unifying and integrating dimension of being that includes the experience of transcendence...and the mystery that is at once overwhelming and fascinating, that renders my existence significant and meaningful in the here and now. It is also a mystery in that it is unmeasurable, unprovable and lacks universal definition.'

So as we reflect upon people with dementia as they confront or experience nature in its many manifestations, can we discern any sense of meaning and purpose, any moments of transcendence that can enable a person to feel significant and meaningful? What Judith Maizels (2010) has described as 'a transcendent doorway to "soul moments"'. Are there experiences which can, in some way, break through their present condition in a meaningful way? I believe that there are and that nature can often be the vehicle for such moments.

---

1   Victor Frankl was a neurologist, psychiatrist and holocaust survivor. His most famous book, *Man's Search for Meaning*, is about his experiences in a concentration camp and how he was able to find meaning even for this.

However, there is a great temptation to think of nature in terms of beauty and benevolence and to ignore its darker side, 'nature red in tooth and claw'. Storms and tempests, aridity, ravenous beasts and death-bearing bacteria. If I have a problem understanding what we mean by spirituality in this context, then I also have a problem with what we mean by nature, recognising the almost inevitable temptation to dwell on the positive aspects and to ignore what might be seen as the harsher or more negative aspects. So this chapter seeks to explore the relationship between two realities which are almost impossible to describe in words.

Kimble, in his definition of spirituality, does not mention religion or God, although many other definitions do. Recognising the validity of the non-religious understanding and experience of spirituality, I shall later move on to the more religious dimension. My references and examples will be Christian in character because that is the tradition in which I have been raised, but I accept that people coming from a different religious tradition will have different but perhaps equally valid experiences, interpretations or stories to tell.

Sally Knocker (2010) tells a wonderful story of sitting with an elderly man in a care home and watching a magnificent sunset. She says that they sat together in silence for fifteen minutes and when the sun had set he turned towards her and said, 'That's what life is all about, isn't it?' She says, 'he was a man with dementia for whom words and clarity of thought were hard to grasp. But in that moment we both felt it and knew.'

Confronting the cosmos can be a daunting task. For some it is a clear, perhaps the clearest argument against any idea of God, whilst for others it leads them into a sense of awe and reverence that speaks to them of God. Coleridge, writing in 1802, writes of his experience of gazing at Mont Blanc:

> ...I gazed upon thee,
> Till thou, still present to the bodily sense,
> Didst vanish from my thought: entranced in prayer
> I worshipped the Invisible alone.
> *Coleridge,* 'Hymn before Sunrise, in the Vale of Chamouni'

The sense of the cosmos having a spiritual nature was well described in a poem by Addison in 1712:

> The spacious firmament on high,
> With all the blue ethereal sky,

And spangled heavens, a shining frame
Their great Original proclaim.
Th'unwearied sun, from day to day,
Does his Creator's powers display,
And publishes to every land
The work of an Almighty Hand.

Soon as the evening shades prevail
The moon takes up the wondrous tale…

In reason's ear they all rejoice,
And utter forth a glorious voice,
Forever singing as they shine,
'The hand that made us is divine.'

Addison, 'The spacious firmament on high'

Modern science has tended to make such assertions unacceptable to a great many people, especially such as expressed in the middle of Addison's poem. Nevertheless, religious or not, the splendour of the universe, often conveyed to us by the beauty of a moonlit night or the wonder of a sunset, can still evoke a sense of awe or wonder. How important it is, therefore, that people with dementia are afforded the opportunity to experience such things. How important it is also that they are able to experience the breeze gently wafting by their face, to be able to smell the flowers and hear the rustling of leaves and the movement of branches and to see the rich variety of birds and other wildlife. Yet a report on care homes with the title *Remember I'm Still Me* (Care Commission and Mental Welfare Commission 2009) stated that, although more than half of the care homes inspected had accessible gardens, there was little evidence of these being used often enough and around half of all people never went out of their care home, so little chance of an encounter with the natural world there then!

A joint venture by Alzheimer's Scotland and Faith in Older People in 2010 produced a DVD, *Spirituality – Have you Found any Yet?* Filmed in a care home in Scotland, it brought together very diverse views from the residents. One lady, being shown a book of photographs of herself taken when she was a very proficient mountaineer, reflected on some of those climbs and commented, 'My mountain climbing days are not over.' The remembrance of those mountains and her climbing exploits brought back to her a sense of her own integrity and meaning and gave her hope and purpose for the future. Another resident reflected on what spirituality meant for her and said, 'Going for a walk makes me feel much better and happier, and I love it.' Two people from the Scottish Dementia Working Group spoke eloquently about their beliefs and how they hoped they would be maintained as their condition deteriorated. Not all that conversation is on the DVD but I felt enormously privileged to be able to explore the issue with them and much of our conversation was about those things which helped to 'raise them out of themselves', and the ability to communicate with nature was central to that conversation. Back in the care home, one particular lady found her identity and purpose in folding napkins. She spoke with immense pride about what she was doing and added, 'and you know, I don't get paid for doing any of this.' Her activity gave her an identity and purpose, which are two parts of Kimble's understanding of spirituality. There was a peacock in the home's grounds and all the residents had their spirits raised when it came near the windows and looked in!

A colleague of mine a few years ago, visiting a resident in a long-stay hospital, one winter's day, created quite a stir when she took in with her a large box full of snow. The lady with dementia being visited was utterly delighted and plunged her hands into the box. Before long snowballs were being thrown to and fro across the ward. It left a bit of a mess, but the sheer delight of those involved made this a memorable and liberating experience. Some would say it was a demonstration of spirituality, a bringing together of people seemingly trapped in their environment with the reality of nature on that winter's day, bringing a sense of joy and wonder, perhaps moments of transcendence.

Different religions have their own ways of exploring the relationship between nature and spirituality, and within the Judaeo-Christian tradition there is a strong link between the two. Creation is seen as an activity of God and the created order often as one of the ways in which people may become aware of the presence of God. There is much in their scriptures to suggest that humankind needs to live harmoniously with the created world, neither exploiting it nor ignoring it. People with dementia who have been brought up within this tradition will possibly or probably be open to all sorts of prompts and cues from nature which may open their selves up to meaning, spiritual understanding and even growth.

The story of the flood and the ensuing rainbow can remind people of the promise of God to be with them forever and never to destroy them. These stories are myths, to be taken not as literal events but as conveying an inner truth. Looking through a dayroom window after a storm and seeing a rainbow may trigger an understanding and a moment of transcendence for a person with dementia. The story of Elijah not finding God in the wind or the fire or the storm but in the still small voice can be a story of insight and support to people who feels themselves to be tossed backwards and forwards by this professional and the other and not knowing where they are. There can be a still small voice which still has power to calm and support. There are many such stories and storytelling has an important part to play in dementia care.

Nature can represent both calmness and beauty or distress and chaos. A few years ago I was having lunch by the Sea of Galilee when, within a matter of minutes, a great storm arose. Tables were thrown about, awnings were ripped and a corrugated roof was blown high into the sky. There is a Biblical story of such a storm and I have used it when talking to someone with dementia who felt that their life was being tossed about and torn apart. The calming of nature can be suggestive of the calming of a person in great distress.

At a much more simplistic level the seasons of the year can help people with dementia to link into their religious tradition. Daffodils mean spring is here, and spring means that Easter is not far away. Autumn brings the expectation of harvest festivals (not in themselves an actual religious festival) and the dark nights of winter herald the coming of Christmas. All people brought up within the Christian tradition and no doubt other religious traditions can point to similar cues.

Two of my friends and former colleagues regularly lead services of worship for people with dementia and what I have observed about these services is that they almost always have an element of nature within them. There are herbs to be passed round and smelt, there are leaves to hold and their different colours to be commented on. There is new-mown grass or hay. I have even seen fish brought in, to be looked at and smelt. Always, it seems, some dialogue with nature. Very often there are pictures projected on a large screen – pictures of the sea, of the hills covered in snow, of lambs or daffodils. I have no idea whether the people attending these services are religious or not, or whether the services are seen as a break in the tedium of the day. My thought, as I have witnessed these services, is that somehow, in helping people to re-connect with nature, what is happening is that an energy is released that can bring both meaning and purpose to people. There is a unifying and integrating process which can, for some people, some time, bring about a moment of transcendence.

We are back to the question of what do we mean by spirituality? I am not wanting to claim that a sense of spirituality has to be connected with some form of religious belief or tradition. Nor am I wanting to claim that some form of religious act or communication is necessarily spiritual in nature. There are many ways in which a 'dialogue with nature' can be, for a person with dementia, a moment of transcendence which many people might call spiritual. Sometimes those moments are religious and spring from an inner faith on the part of the person with dementia, or they are in some way communicated or enabled by another person who has some form of faith – and often they are not. Returning to my original definition by Mel Kimble, such experiences are a mystery that are unmeasurable, unprovable and lack a universal definition, but even so they can be real and life-enhancing.

References

Addison, J. (1672–1719) 'The Spacious firmament on high.' In D. Davie (ed.) (1981) *The New Oxford Book of Christian Verse.* Oxford: Oxford University Press.

Care Commission and Mental Welfare Commission (2009) *Remember I'm Still Me.* Edinburgh: Mental Welfare Commission.

Coleridge, S.T. (1772–1834) 'Hymn before Sunrise, in the Vale of Chamouni.' Available at www.poetryfoundation.org/poem/173244, accessed on 15 September 2011.

Faith in Older People (2010) *Spirituality – Have you Found any Yet?* [DVD] Available at www.faithinolderpeople.org.uk/dvds-and-cds/4533949596, accessed on 15 September 2011.

Kimble, M. (2001) 'A Personal Journey of Aging: The Spiritual Dimension.' In S.H. McFadden and R.C. Atchley (eds) *Aging and the Meaning of Time.* New York: Springer Publishing Co.

Knocker, S. (2010) 'Snapshots in Time.' In J. Gilliard and M. Marshall (eds) *Time for Dementia.* London: Hawker Publications.

Maizels, J. (2010) 'A Transcendent Doorway to "Soul Moments".' In J. Gilliard and M. Marshall (eds) *Time for Dementia.* London: Hawker Publications.

Chapter 2

Sunlight and Daylight

DAVID MCNAIR

It's not 'natural' for humans to be confined indoors. From an evolutionary perspective, man is not a creature that should spend significant time periods indoors. *Homo sapiens* originated some 100,000 to 2.5 million years ago in Africa as a primitive hunter gatherer. By the start of the industrial revolution in the late eighteenth century, man had evolved and was using quite sophisticated farming methods, but the majority of daylight hours were still spent outdoors. As a consequence, it is reasonable to assume that human biological systems evolved accordingly. For example, the benefits of light to health were demonstrated during the industrial revolution when smoke from factories reduced the amount of daylight reaching ground level, causing an epidemic of rickets in industrial cities throughout Europe. Rickets is a condition where lack of vitamin D causes bones to soften, deform and potentially fracture. Exposure to sunlight was found to be a ready cure. Current research indicates that the number and severity of falls is also reduced with good levels of vitamin D (see the following section).

Exposure to daylight also helps regulate the circadian (internal biological) rhythms, resulting in improved sleep and patient health. High levels of light, particularly in the winter when natural levels are low, can contribute to a reduced incidence of seasonal affective disorder and make everyone happier. Therapeutic views from buildings can reduce stress but why not experience them first hand? The message is 'get outdoors'.

Vitamin D

For vitamin D to be manufactured in the body there has to be skin exposure to direct sunlight, rather than just daylight, and at UK latitudes the sunlight only has sufficient power to trigger the process between April and September inclusive.

Adequate levels of vitamin D are very good at reducing falls in older people. It works by maximizing calcium and phosphorous absorption, which improves bone growth, and lowering levels of hormone that would otherwise decrease bone density and weaken muscles. A research project (Bischoff-Ferrari *et al.* 2009) that analysed many trials revealed that levels of vitamin D above a daily intake of 700 IU[1] reduced falls by between 19 and 26 per cent and concluded that a daily intake is warranted in all people over 65. It was also found that below this threshold of 700 IU daily, the vitamin produced no effect.

Researchers have identified an *association* between low levels of vitamin D and various diseases such as colorectal cancer, cardiovascular disease and multiple sclerosis, in addition to mood disorder and impaired cognitive performance. This association means that, while a vitamin D shortfall has been identified, it cannot yet be proven whether the disease causes the shortfall or the shortfall causes the disease. Perhaps the solution to this conundrum came closer when in 2010 genome researchers identified that vitamin D receptor binding sites were particularly numerous near genes that had previously been identified as being linked to autoimmune diseases and cancer. The theory is that pathogens in the bloodstream are not able to bind to the genes because the vitamin D binds first. As the pathogens cannot bind, they cannot disrupt the genes to cause disease and the chances of them being destroyed by antioxidants increases. The possible link to melatonin, an extremely efficient free radical scavenger that is produced overnight, should be noted.

Vitamin D can be obtained from food, supplements or exposure to sunlight, with the latter being extremely effective. It has been found that low consumption of fish is linked to reduced vitamin D levels. A daily amount of 3000 IU of Vitamin D, if achieved even every second day in the summer, would be sufficient to tide a person over the winter. For comparison purposes this dose of 3000 IU can be obtained by eating ten tins of sardines or 150 egg yolks or 210 ounces (almost 6 kilograms) of butter or by spending, on average, five to ten minutes with arms and legs exposed to direct sunlight (at UK latitudes). The quoted time period of five to ten minutes varies with latitude and time of year, less exposure being needed at lower latitudes and in midsummer. Non-smokers, younger people and those with lighter skin all need less exposure than their opposites. Of course there is a trade-off because burning of the skin can lead to malignant melanoma, a type of cancer; however, sensible exposure to the sun, avoiding burning, is beneficial.

However, it should be noted that in 2010 there were many reports that rickets is making a comeback in British children who only go outdoors

---

1   International units. For vitamin D, 1 IU equals 25 x 10^{-9}g or 0.025μg.

with factor 50 sunscreen applied. Also worthy of consideration is that British people with hereditary dark skin are more susceptible to vitamin D deficiency. In addition, some researchers have postulated that light skin evolved to safeguard the mother/child unit by reducing the risk of pelvic rickets by ensuring sufficient production of vitamin D in populations that have migrated from tropical areas. Nevertheless it is important to take precaution to avoid reddening of the skin, and in this regard some may be happier with the application of factor eight sunscreen – but this increases the necessary average time exposure to about 140 minutes. Perhaps if people go outdoors to apply their sunscreen, they will have achieved most of the desired exposure by the time the sunscreen is applied.

A further benefit of exposure to sunlight has been noted through the ages, namely its ability to kill various bacteria.

People should always wear sunglasses when exposed to direct sunlight to minimise the risk of damage to the eyes.

Circadian rhythm

The body's internal biological clock, its circadian rhythm, is very important in contributing to good quality sleep and adequate energy levels. Elderly people have more frequent wakenings than the young, and reduced rapid eye movement sleep, which is important for memory. Researchers have postulated that at least in part this is due to disruption of the circadian rhythm. In people with Alzheimer's disease the changes greatly exceed those of normal ageing, contributing to fatigue and further cognitive impairment. In addition increased nocturnal activity has been noted, hardly surprising if people cannot sleep. A delay in the circadian rhythm of temperature has been identified as an important factor. On a positive note it has been identified that exposure to high morning light levels produces a beneficial impact by training the circadian rhythms, which in turn improves sleep efficiency, reduces waking time at night by up to two hours, reduces behavioural disturbance, and indeed improves nursing staff ratings in care environments. A minimum figure of 5000 lux hours is believed to produce the desired effect, although some claim it is as high as 16,000 lux hours. Taking an average of 10,000 lux hours this can be achieved by exposing people to 10,000 lux for one hour, 5000 lux for two hours, or any equivalent combination. As the average light level in a lounge area is about 300 lux (although the Dementia Services Development Centre at the University of Stirling recommends 600 lux; McNair, Cunningham, Pollock and McGuire 2010) a period of nearly 33 hours would be required to achieve this indoors. The alternatives, in increasing order of preference, are as follows:

1. Have a very bright room with the necessary large number of lights to provide the light. This is an expensive option both in terms of installation and running costs.

2. Have people sit one metre from a light box for about one hour. There are difficulties related to sitting for this period and discomfort from the bright light so close to the face. An additional difficulty in care environments concerns the number of light boxes available.

3. Have internal space(s) where there is significant daylight penetration; this would be within about two metres of reasonably large windows or glass doors.

4. Go outdoors, where light levels are very much higher than indoors with an illumination that will barely drop below 15,000 lux in mid-morning throughout the year in the UK. Unlike the requirement for production of vitamin D in the body, direct sunlight is not essential and a clear or even overcast sky is sufficient. One hour outdoors daily will therefore easily deliver even the highest possible requirement. When the sun is shining the necessary light exposure can even be obtained while under covered outdoor spaces. Again, it is best to wear sunglasses when exposed to direct sunlight. However, again unlike the production of vitamin D, it is light into the eye that is important; if the sun is sufficiently bright to require sunglasses, then there will be sufficient light to help regulate the circadian rhythms. Likewise if there is no direct sun and no sunglasses are worn, there will be sufficient light.

The detectors in the eye that detect the light to activate the biological clock are more sensitive to (short wavelength) blue light than longer wavelengths. The colour of the sky varies through the day, being bluer in the morning and redder towards evening. It is plausible that lighting systems that mimic this by producing a bluer light in the morning and a redder light in late afternoon will produce a beneficial impact on circadian rhythm. However, a host of research projects have found that this wavelength (colour) change is not required if there is sufficient exposure to daylight in the first place.

Many researchers have suggested that morning exposure to bright light can contribute to a reduction in the incidence of 'sundowning', a condition where people with dementia become irritable in the evening. This is plausible because the bright light suppresses the production of the (sleep) hormone melatonin and promotes the production of the (activity) hormone serotonin and this contributes to a proper sleep regime, i.e. overnight. A further contribution to this appropriate sleep regime is achieved by making sure that bedrooms are dark overnight, as light at that time would suppress the melatonin production that helps sleep and neutralises pathogens in the body.

This suggested exposure to light helps carers by reducing the waking occurrences of people with dementia, at the same time as improving the quality of the carer's sleep.

Seasonal affective disorder

Seasonal affective disorder (SAD) is a type of depression that leaves people tired, lethargic, stressed and unhappy, with mood, appetite and energy levels affected. It tends to appear when the days are shorter, dark and gloomy, with symptoms usually disappearing in spring. Up to one in eight people in the UK experiences at least mild symptoms of sub-syndromal SAD (sub-SAD).

People tend to associate the prevalence of SAD and sub-SAD with increased latitude. However, the research does not entirely support this association and has found that climate, genetic vulnerability and social-cultural context are important factors and that diagnosis is not without problems. Studies comparing the incidence in different continents (Mersch et al. 1999) found it to be twice as high in the USA as in Europe, whereas the opposite would be expected since the latitudes used in the European studies were higher.

On the other hand, a highly positive correlation with cloudiness has been found (Potkin et al. 1986), together with significant correlations between mood and minutes of sunshine, length of daylight and temperature.

A study of Icelandic descendants in Canada found the rate of winter SAD was nearer the lower rate of Iceland compared to the higher rate of Canada, leading to speculation about genetic adaptation playing a role, or the influence of omega-3 essential fatty acids from fish in the diet (and as an extension vitamin D). A similar and unexpected previous finding of low prevalence of SAD in Japan, which also has a high per capita intake of fish, was noted. However, Japan also has a cultural predisposition not to express complaints that might be perceived to demonstrate 'weakness'. One study in Montgomery County, Maryland, in the USA found a 50 per cent higher rate of SAD than one in the same location during the previous year. It is unfortunate that the authors did not investigate whether or not weather conditions differed in the years studied. Several studies have shown that between 60 per cent and 74 per cent of people diagnosed with SAD did not have the condition several years later (see list in Mersch *et al.* 1999).

Exposure to light has been found to be an effective agent for relieving the symptoms of SAD and sub-SAD. As typical exposures quoted are between 5000 and 10,000 lux hours daily, the prognosis becomes that shown above for regulation of the circadian rhythm. Similarly, the most effective time of the day for treatment is described as during the morning, and this may be because the bright light suppresses the production of the (sleep) hormone melatonin and promotes the production of the (activity) hormone serotonin.

Therapeutic views

Many studies (e.g. Ulrich 1984, 2002) have found that people prefer natural rather than urban views for the buildings they occupy. Researchers have identified many benefits of this preference: shorter recovery times and reduced analgesic intake for surgical patients; reduced stress in hospital patients; a similar reduction in stress of office workers; and higher staff satisfaction in health care environments. Now, some people will have lovely natural views and others will not. In either case the easiest way of combining a natural view with the benefits of daylight and exercise may be to take a short walk to the local park, a river walkway, a canal bank, or the tearoom at a local garden centre.

Summary

So, in summary, exposure to even short periods of sunlight helps produce vitamin D in the body and this has various positive effects for health: reduction in the number and severity of falls and potentially reduced susceptibility to some diseases.

In addition, exposure to bright morning light triggers a burst of energy that makes people active, at the same time contributing to good quality sleep by training the circadian rhythms and reducing the incidence of symptoms of seasonal depression. Daylight does this job just as well as sunlight. If this exposure to light is achieved by taking external exercise, even if only pottering about in the garden, this further aids the quality of sleep. Being outside in itself has a therapeutic effect. In addition sunlight kills some types of bacteria, and colds and flu-like viruses are spread less easily than in internal spaces because of the superior air flow.

All the benefits stated here have a double impact on carers: directly by improving their own sleep and health, and indirectly by impacting on the sleep and health of the people they are looking after.

References

Bischoff-Ferrari, H.A., Dawson-Hughes, B., Staehelin, H.B., Orav, J.E. *et al.* (2009) 'Fall prevention with supplemental and active forms of vitamin D: a meta-analysis of randomised controlled trials.' *British Medical Journal 339,* b3692.

McNair, D., Cunningham, C., Pollock, R. and McGuire, B. (2010) *Light and Lighting Design for People With Dementia.* Stirling: The Dementia Services Development Centre, University of Stirling.

Mersch, P.P.A., Middendorp, H.M. *et al.* (1999) 'Seasonal affective disorder and latitude: A review of the literature.' *Journal of Affective Disorders 53,* 35–48.

Potkin, S.G., Zetin, M., Stamenkovic, V. *et al.* (1986) 'Seasonal affective disorder: Prevalence varies with latitude climate.' *Clinical Neuropharmacology 9,* 181–183.

Ulrich, R.S. (1984) 'View through a window may influence recovery from surgery.' *Science 224,* 420–421.

Ulrich, R.S. (2002) 'Health benefits of gardens in hospitals.' Seminar presented at the International Exhibition Floriade, Haarlemmerme, the Netherlands.

Chapter 3

Living with Dementia through the Changing Seasons

NEIL MAPES

Introduction

Dementia is a term we are now hearing ever more frequently both in our families and communities and in the media. There is a common narrative which few of us have escaped in recent times that the numbers of people living with dementia is increasing dramatically. The Alzheimer's Society estimate that there are roughly 750,000 people in the UK with some form of dementia, with about 16,000 people under the age of 65 (Alzheimer's Society 2010). One in 14 people over the age of 65, and one in six people over the age of 80, has a form of dementia (Alzheimer's Society 2010). The total number of people living with dementia in the UK is forecast to increase to nearly a million in the next ten years (Alzheimer's Society 2007), and this is arguably a conservative estimate. Whilst these figures are potentially both daunting and depressing in equal measure, genuine hope remains for a scientific breakthrough, but it is frustrating that this breakthrough feels too far off in the future for the many thousands of people living with dementia, who want changes now.

What we can change is our understanding and approach to dementia, both individually and collectively. This change involves a shift from connecting with each other primarily on a cognitive level (with our cognitive intelligence), to connecting from the heart (emotional intelligence). There is something deeply personal and emotional about our connection with nature and with the changing of the seasons, and our human well-being depends on it. The seasons are a continuous and unending cycle which we can connect with and witness simply by the act of getting outdoors and by having contact with nature. The seasons remind us that change is universal, and so are a helpful starting place for us to consider how we can change the way dementia is currently understood and enable more people to live well with dementia.

The seasons have been the subject of all of our cultural and creative endeavours, have been interpreted in a multitude of ways and have fascinated us for millennia. 'The Seasons' has been the title of classical music (Tchaikovsky's), dance (Jean-Baptiste Lully's ballet) and literature (*The Seasons* by James Thompson) and perhaps the most well known, 'The Four Seasons' by Vivaldi. In Hong Kong there is even a TV drama called 'The Seasons'. In Greek mythology the *Horae* were the goddesses of the seasons, the natural portions of time. They were originally the personifications of nature in its different seasonal aspects. Traditionally the aboriginal people of Australia defined the seasons by what was happening to the plants, animals and weather around them. This led to each separate tribal group having different seasons, some with up to eight seasons each year.

Ancient Celts divided the seasons into summer and winter, these being marked by the festivals of *Beltaine* and *Samhain*. In the Hindu calendar there are six seasons or *Ritu*. Chinese seasons are traditionally based on 24 periods known as *solar terms*. In tropical climates there is the monsoon and the dry season, while cold regions have 'polar day' (spring and summer) and 'polar night' (autumn and winter). *Longyearbyen* in Norway is the northernmost town on the planet and consequently gets four months of darkness each winter; it is now the focus of a study by electrical appliance company Philips, who are looking at the benefits of waking up to light called 'Wake up the town' (Grush 2010). Different parts of the world have 'hurricane season' or 'wildfire season', there are breeding and growing seasons for animals and plants, and don't forget the 'silly season' – for example, when April Fools stories make the media.

However, in the UK and for many Western cultures our tradition is of the four changing seasons of spring, summer, autumn and winter. Also the notion of the seasons changing in a cycle or a circle is a common thread across cultures (however many seasons there may be in each cultural interpretation). This is not surprising, given that the world itself is round and indeed, as John Ruskin's nineteenth-century prose reminds us, 'nature is all made up of roundnesses; not the roundness of perfect globes, but of variously curved surfaces' (Ruskin 1876). Contact with and connection with nature simply, yet profoundly, connects us to something whole, to the seasons, to a universal pattern of change, and to a cycle of life bigger than our own individual existence.

Changing seasons

I believe human well-being depends on contact with nature. Kaplan said that the natural world satisfies our need for contemplation, escape, restoration and distraction (Kaplan 1995). Once a person receives a diagnosis and label of dementia they appear to be at increased risk of not being able to get out into nature. This pattern of decreasing opportunity and decreasing connection with the natural world also appears proportionally to get worse as the disease progresses. This is often simply because of an increasingly risk-averse culture combined with a poor understanding of dementia. Witnessing the seasons and experiencing the benefits this brings can quickly become out of reach for many people living with dementia, particularly if there are other complicating physical health issues. Yet this is clearly counter to what we intuitively know – that nature is good for us. If there was ever a time for contemplation, escape, restoration and distraction, then surely having a life-changing illness is the time. The physical act of getting out into nature, witnessing seasonal changes, is important, but the changing seasons also allow us to reflect on our own changes, on our own lives.

Norman McNamara is a gentleman, blogger and activist (and is living with early onset Alzheimer's). He shares his thoughts and experiences online and has kindly agreed to share a piece of his writing called 'Changing Colours of the Seasons'. His words tell us a great deal about what the seasons mean to him currently.

Changing Colours of the Seasons

I couldn't imagine living anywhere else in the world with the glorious changing colours of the seasons. I was gazing at these wonderful views on my way to Budleigh Salterton this morning when I started to think about how the seasons are very similar to life itself and the connection with Alzheimer's disease.

Spring is like our births when the newborn flowers and the rebirth of others push through the soil and are there for all to see with their fresh and young shoots growing rapidly into something quite beautiful.

Summer is all about things growing up and turning into adulthood whilst showing off their wonderful coats and colours, becoming mature and settled. Autumn is as we get older and things start to change. This is also the season that reminds me of my illness the most. As the trees and landscapes change their colours so do we with this awful illness and things seem to take on a different meaning. The leaves slowly but surely decay and start to look a shadow of their former selves. But as with anything all is not lost. If you look very closely, beyond the falling leaves and into the landscape, you can still see the same beauty and soul that lives on within all of us. We are still here, as are the trees and fields, and we still need looking after and nurturing as do all living things. Unfortunately along comes the bleakness of winter (late stages of AD) when nothing seems to grow anymore and the landscape seems to fall silent. This is the worst time of all, especially for the nature lovers (carers) who just want things to get back to normal and the fields and trees to blossom again. But as we know, they sadly cannot during winter.

I hope you have all enjoyed this little walk through the seasons with me, and even though it may seem a sad one, always remember the three seasons before winter and all it entails as these memories will hopefully stay with you forever. (McNamara 2010)

An interesting reply to this web posting was, 'Even in the middle of winter, there are the most surprisingly bright and beautiful days, Norm.' The poet Shelley asked, 'If winter comes, can spring be far behind?' And so we begin this philosophical and practical discussion about the importance of the changing seasons to people living with dementia. In discovering Norman's posting I was struck by his phrase 'we are still here, as are the trees and fields...' Professor John Zeisel's recent book is entitled *I'm Still Here: A Breakthrough Approach to Understanding Someone Living with Alzheimer's.* Zeisel writes:

> It is likely that the need for contact with the natural environment and the feelings we have about nature and being outdoors are hardwired, partly because this is the source of our food. Sunshine, flowers, shade, moonlight, and trees are all so much a part of our basic nature that no one has to be taught to respond to such stimuli. Again, not surprisingly, gardens and nature are much appreciated by those with this illness. (Zeisel 2009)

I would argue that it is our frequent contact with and connection with nature that also connects us with the rhythm of the changing seasons. Dementia appears, subjectively at least, to disrupt or halt this natural cycle. A second online contribution entitled 'When Autumn comes early' was posted by Bruce Bane, who lives in Iowa in the USA. His blog site is called 'Living With Dementia', where he publicly shares his reflections on how dementia affects his life and relationships, and he has agreed to share this piece of writing. Bruce, who is living with frontotemporal dementia, asks, 'How can I see this season of dementia?'

When Autumn Comes Early

'There is a time for everything, and a season for every activity under heaven.' (*Ecclesiastes* 3:1)

I have thought about this verse a lot lately, especially as I watch the seasons changing. The seasons of nature are predictable, coming and going at just the right time. And each season has its own purpose. But when I think about the seasons of my life it seems that autumn has come too early and winter is fast approaching. This is dementia's doing. The season of dementia came early for me and it is unpredictable. What I do know is that this early autumn will lead to an early winter and that will be the last season. This is dementia's time, dementia's season in my life and there is no undoing this.

But reading further in Chapter 3 of *Ecclesiastes* I found this: '(God) has made everything beautiful in its time' (*Ecclesiastes* 3:11). Everything is made beautiful in its time... What is made beautiful in this time of dementia? Surely this doesn't mean that dementia is beautiful! So where is the beauty? What does God see that I can't? Maybe a better question is 'How can I see this season of dementia and decline through God's eyes; eyes that focus on what is beautiful?' I don't have any answers, but these are questions I need to keep asking. They are challenging, but I also think they might be a way to help me through the dark times that I experience. (Bane 2010)

The experience of dementia like the seasons being broken, or autumn and winter coming too early, gives us an insight into living with dementia that is profound. Bruce is asking questions which are extremely important. Put slightly differently, how can we see the beauty of spring when we are engulfed by the darkness of winter? In literature we may look for answers, particularly the references to the seasons as circles. In writing this chapter I was reminded of the work of the writings of Black Elk. He tells us:

Everything the Power of the World does is done in a circle. The sky is round, and I have heard that the earth is round like a ball, and so are all the stars. The wind, in its greatest power, whirls. Birds make their nests in circles, for theirs is the same religion as ours. The sun comes forth and goes down again in a circle. The moon does the same, and both are round. Even the seasons form a great circle in their changing, and always come back again to where they were. The life of a man is a circle from childhood to childhood, and so it is in everything where power moves. (Neihardt 2004)

To quote a line from Shakespeare's *Hamlet*: 'They say an old man is twice a child' (Act 2, Scene 2, 380–1). Many centuries before Shakespeare in the fifth century BC Aristophanes said, 'Men are children twice over.' For me these references in literature remind us of a beauty yet to come, like the spring we cannot yet see.

Returning to John Zeisel, he has a chapter in his book called 'The Gifts of Alzheimer's', which could also be called 'the beauty of Alzheimer's'. In this he shares some beautiful insights gained from learning to give and receive and be together with people living with dementia. The chapter is wonderful in sharing 'gifts' in a way many have yet to consider. The one I most relate to is the 'gift of enjoying the moment' in which a carer shares this:

My mother is perpetually in the moment. Whenever we are together, I am given the cherished gift of being there with her at that moment. Any regrets about the past I might have, or hopes or fears about the future, have little place in our relationship at that moment. The feeling of being present to life lingers on long after we have been together. (Zeisel 2009)

Georgina Noakes is a remarkable lady, using poetry is corporate settings. We met recently and were discussing the significance for all of us in 'truly being in' and 'enjoying the moment'. I was relating to her the wonderful moments which occur when people living with dementia connect with something in nature, an aspect of the current season (e.g. new ducklings on the river). In these moments we are in harmony, for a moment the dementia isn't there, just a person gazing at the beauty of a fluffy baby duckling starting out in life. Georgina was inspired to write 'Walking through the seasons', which again takes us through the seasons but this time with the beauty of the present moment in mind, and has kindly agreed to share it here.

Walking through the seasons

Take my hand and walk with me.
Here
and now
beneath a clear spring sky.

Stay with me
whilst I stop to watch a dance of daffodils
nodding to a blackbird's song.

Here I feel the grass singing beneath my feet.
Now is where I can be.
You have found me, caught in the present,
no pull of the past, no promise of the future.

Here there are no more yesterdays or tomorrows.
Now there's no time like the present to bring me joy.
As long as I can see the trees I shall be happy,
the changing seasons caught in their sway.

Stay with me as spring grows into summer,
soft rose petals, caught like velvet
between my finger and thumb.

Stay with me.
Here is the reward of today,
with no fear of tomorrow or regret from yesterday.

The swallows fly to where I can now never go
taking the last of the summer sun upon their wings.
Stay with me as I walk through autumn,
falling leaves like my lost memories trodden crisply under
    foot.

Here I feel alive, the breeze across my face.
Now is where I will spend my days.
And it is where you will find me, caught in the present,
no pull of the past, no promise of the future.

Here there are no more yesterdays or tomorrows.
Now there's no time like the present to bring me joy.

See with fresh eyes how winter arrives.
Feel the frost caressing branch and fern alike.

Touch my hot breath hanging in the air
like early morning mist rising over newly ploughed fields.
My ruddy cheeks warm beneath a woollen hat.

Through my eyes you will see such wonder.
Savour the smell of the earth.
Walk with me and watch the silent snow fall
like a new miracle.

Stay here as I am held, spellbound, by this one perfect
moment.

Georgina Noakes, November 2010
(Written for Dementia Adventure)

Changing understanding

Georgina was inspired by Dementia Adventure. I lead Dementia
Adventure, a small social enterprise providing adventure travel and short
breaks for people living with dementia. We have a vision of society
in which people live well with dementia, are connected to nature and
enjoy a sense of adventure. When people are connected with nature their
dementia often takes a back step and becomes less of a focus. Forward
steps a human being in the moment of nature. Nature plays to the
strengths of people living with dementia (emotional memory), not their
weaknesses (cognition) – you do not need to 'remember' the beauty of an
apple tree in full blossom. Dementia Adventure is connecting with more
and more people who wish to stay connected to nature and the changing
seasons. I recently went walking with Brian, a man living with dementia
who goes out walking every day of the year. He said that walking out
in nature helped 'dampen down the symptoms' of his dementia (Mapes
2011).

In March 2010, Dementia Adventure teamed up with Innovations in
Dementia CIC to enjoy a walk around the house and gardens of Standen
(a National Trust property) with a group of people living with dementia.
One of the gentleman remarked, 'When I walk around looking at these
things, I forget I have dementia.' I remain struck by the simplicity and
beauty of this statement. Often we look for complicated solutions, we
try to 'fix' people and things, rather than seeing the simple solution.
Perhaps we can 'do' less and 'be' together more. Often the environments
in which people living with dementia find themselves are both indoors
and characterised by 'doing', and are often necessarily 'task-focused',

with little room for 'just being together' out in nature. Our connection with the changing seasons is so fundamental, we seem to have almost overlooked it or been distracted away from it. We as a society have yet to answer fully the question: What does it look and feel like to live well with dementia? I would argue that it is the simple act of contact with nature and its changing seasons that is an essential element in living and feeling well with dementia.

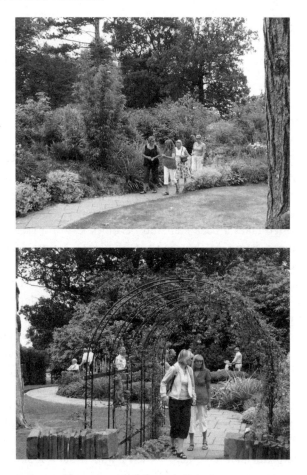

Figure 3.1 'Walk and Talk Together' in the gardens of Hylands House (event organised by Dementia Adventure)
Photos: Neil Mapes

I have been spending an increasing amount of my time in parks and green spaces recently and enabling people living with dementia and their carers to do the same. Green spaces are largely a free community resource. Even in the city you are often not too far from a small green space. Yet how often do we think of these places as therapeutic places for people living with dementia? In what way can we enable people living with dementia to live a beautiful life right now – in nature, with the seasons? Not in ten years' time with the promise of a new wonder drug. In what way can we be together outside in nature?

In the autumn and winter of 2010 Dementia Adventure scheduled six weekly walks called 'Walk and Talk Together'. These events were held in beautiful parks and woodlands across Essex. We woke on the morning of one of the walks to find that nearly six inches of snow had fallen overnight. I spoke with the support worker for a lady in her 80s living with dementia, who was due to come on the walk. Much to my pleasure the lady told her support worker, 'I am definitely still going out.' This lady may well be part of a growing group of people living with dementia who know that nature helps them and do all they can to get out into nature every day. I recently went on a three-hour ramble across the fields with a gentleman living with dementia in Essex, for whom the walk was very much his therapy. Indeed, his dementia-related symptoms were much less significant on our walk than when we were in his house together. In particular he was much more verbally fluent on the walk.

In July 2010 Dementia Adventure organised three 'Walk and Talk Together' events in the majestic park of Hylands House in Essex. We spent time with over 50 people living with dementia, their carers and supporters, both in the historic house and strolling around the grounds and gardens stopping to share history and revel in the beauty of the nature in front of us (see Figure 3.1). One of the ladies who attended the event did so in a wheelchair being pushed by her husband. I had previously listened to this man telling me about her challenging behaviour and how difficult things were at home. It had been a big emotional step for them to join our walk. The lady was full of joy and smiled for almost the entire walk and appeared to revel in the closeness to nature. At these events people shared their thoughts and feedback on their Dementia Adventure, saying:

'Just offering opportunities to get out of the house means a lot to people.'

'She thoroughly enjoyed the day, the brightest she's been for a long time.'

'It was nice to get out and see kids running around the gardens.'

'It is about exercise and beauty, isn't it?'

'Thank you for being brave and taking this on.'

'Difficult to find the motivation to do stuff other than day centres.'

'It is important to get out and talk to people.'

'The first time it is difficult but at the end of the day you think that was worth it.'

'Activity, fresh air, stimulation, being together as a group.'

The benefits of these events showed that people living with dementia were more verbally fluent and generally instigated more communication when on the nature walk than when in the house (Mapes 2010). People had a tangible and obvious sense of joy and sensory pleasure, such as from sitting on a bench in the sunshine looking at the flowers. But people also got to make friends and talk to each other in a way that was not forced or uncomfortable, both characteristics some carers identified with some support group settings they had previously experienced. Getting out into nature, getting fresh air and exercise were all important to people, as well as meeting and talking to other people. People felt safer going as a group who were 'all in the same boat' and understood dementia. This has implications for all kinds of engagement exercises, for support groups and Alzheimer cafés, and indeed in any setting where people living with dementia come together.

There is a well-proven bank of evidence which confirms what we implicitly already know – that 'the natural environment is good for us'. Julie Newton's general overview of the evidence on well-being and the natural environment (Newton 2007) provides an example for the interested reader. It is well known that exposure to natural places leads to better mental health whether it be a view from a window (Ulrich 1984), being in nature (Pretty *et al.* 2005) or exercising in these spaces (Pretty *et al.* 2007). There are clear benefits to activity in nature for a wide variety of people. These benefits include improved self-esteem and improved mood, and often these benefits can be experienced from as little as five minutes out in nature, particularly where there is water (Barton and Pretty 2010). Chalfont's research showed how connection to nature can enhance verbal expression in people living with dementia (Chalfont 2006). Chalfont identified that nature-based activities for people living with dementia bring joy and sensory stimulation. He also found that family and professional carers play an important role in enabling a person living with dementia to maintain a connection to nature by overcoming obstacles.

Dementia Adventure is attracting an increasing number of followers for our work in getting people out into nature. People in India, Canada and Japan have all connected with our simple message 'nature is good for you'. The overriding message we have learnt the last 18 months or so in talking to people living with dementia about Dementia Adventure is 'don't delay, we need this today' – there is a sense of urgency for those living with dementia, five or ten years for scientific breakthroughs can feel like a lifetime away for many. The onus is on us all working in this field to get started, to support people to get out into nature, witnessing the beauty of the changing moments of the seasons. Getting out into nature is of course not without its problems, with getting cold, wet, falling over and traffic dangers to consider, amongst others. We may rate these risks much higher than people living with dementia. Often the person living with dementia is more concerned about their loss of self, of self-worth, and self-identity.

Work like that by Jones and Van der Eerden (2008) is important in highlighting the potential complexities of people living with dementia positively benefiting from being active in nature. Their work focuses on visual perceptual considerations, such as glare in bright sunshine, the potential illusion effects of shadows and reflective surfaces, which all need our careful attention – for example, in walking around lakes in the summer. The benefits of the activities should also be just as carefully considered as the risks. There may be significant benefits in terms of physical health (e.g. better mobility) and psychological health (e.g. sense of worth and identity) which outweigh the risks of a 'dementia adventure' in nature. For more on risk/benefit and dementia, readers are directed to the Nuffield Council on Bioethics report (2009).

Conclusion

Norman and Bruce are not alone in their need for contemplation, escape and restoration. The changing seasons of our year and the changing seasons of our lives are all part of a universal pattern of change. Physical contact with and connection with the seasons offers all of us an opportunity to be part of nature, to feel and live well. If we can see the changes of the seasons, we can see the change in ourselves. The physical and philosophical connections with the seasons are of equal importance in addressing this illness called dementia. The increase in the numbers of people living with dementia could easily be compared to winter approaching too early with not enough resources to go round. If we view dementia through nature's lens, if we think less with our heads and feel more with our hearts, then a new, more positive understanding can emerge. Like a bright sunny day in winter, dementia can bring us gifts and beauty. From the depths of winter spring does eventually come. It is essential that we change the way we understand dementia, in a shift from the cognitive to the emotional, from 'doing to' to 'being with', and strive to find ways to enable our deeply personal and emotional connection with nature to remain in the presence of advancing dementia.

References

Alzheimer's Society (2007) *Dementia UK 2007*. London: Alzheimer's Society.

Alzheimer's Society (2010) *Demographic Information*. Accessed at www.alzheimers.org.uk on 27 July 2010.

Bane, B (2010) 'When autumn comes early.' Living with Dementia, Iowa USA. Author website: www.brucebane.wordpress.com.

Barton, J. and Pretty, J. (2010) 'What is the best dose of nature and green exercise for improving mental health? A multi-study analysis.' *Environmental Science and Technology 44*, 10, 3947–3955.

Chalfont, G. (2006) 'Connection to Nature at the Building Edge: Towards a Therapeutic Architecture for Dementia Care Environments.' PhD thesis. University of Sheffield.

Grush, L. (2010) 'Town in perpetual night receives ultimate night lights.' Published by FoxNews.com on 4 November 2010.

Jones, G.M.M. and van der Eerden, W.J. (2008) 'Designing care environments for persons with Alzheimer's disease: Visuoperceptual considerations.' Review in *Clinical Gerontology 18*, 13–37.

Kaplan, S. (1995) 'The restorative benefits of nature: Towards an integrative framework.' *Journal of Environmental Psychology 15*, 3 169–182.

McNamara, N. (2010) 'Changing colours of the seasons.' Author website: www.norrms. web.officelive.com.

Mapes, N. (2011) 'Living with dementia and connecting with nature – looking back and stepping forwards.' Essex: Dementia Adventure. Research available at www. dementiaadventure.co.uk.

Mapes, N. (2010) 'It's a walk in the park: Exploring the benefits of green exercise and open spaces for people living with dementia.' *Working with Older People 14*, 4, 25–31.

Neihardt, J.G. (2004) *Black Elk Speaks*. Lincoln and London: University of Nebraska Press.

Newton, J. (2007) *Wellbeing and the Natural Environment: A Brief Overview of the Evidence.* London: Department of Environment, Food and Rural Affairs.

Noakes, G. (2010) 'Walking through the seasons.' Author website: www.brightsideoflife. co.uk.

Nuffield Council on Bioethics (2009) *Dementia: Ethical Issues.* Cambridge: Cambridge Publishers.

Pretty, J., Peacock, J., Hine, R., Sellens, M., South, N. and Griffin, M. (2007) 'Green exercise in the UK countryside: Effects on health and psychological well-being, and implications for policy and planning.' *Journal of Environmental Planning and Management 50,* 2, 211–231.

Pretty, J., Peacock, J., Sellens, M. and Griffin, M. (2005) 'The mental and physical health outcomes of green exercise.' *International Journal Of Environmental Health Research 15,* 5, 319–337.

Ruskin, J. (1876) *The Elements of Drawing: In Three Letters to Beginners.* New York: John Wiley and Sons. Republished Bernard Dustan (ed.) (1991) London: The Herbert Press.

Thompson, J. (1981) *The Seasons,* edited with introduction and commentary by James Sambrook. Oxford: Clarendon Press.

Ulrich, R.S. (1984) 'View through a window may influence recovery from surgery.' *Science 224,* 420–421.

Zeisel, J. (2009) *I'm Still Here: A Breakthrough Approach to Understanding Someone Living with Alzheimer's.* New York: Penguin.

Chapter 4

The Forget Me Not Centre

LYNDA HUGHES

I have been presenting Ramblings for over ten years and over that time, a few programmes really stand out as being exceptional. My walk with the Forget Me Not ramblers was, for me, at the top of that list. So many people who listened to the programme said that they had never heard people with Alzheimer's talking at such length about what it meant to live with the disease.

It was so revealing to talk about the different stages of Alzheimer's, to discuss methods that help people cope – such as wearing a bright red T-shirt so that when you got lost, you could be found and taken home. I also felt that the Forget Me Nots were harnessing the healing power of walking and using it to their advantage. It is a non-threatening, non-competitive activity which encourages people to read a map, find their way, talk to others and share an experience.

I have read academic research into the mental health benefits of walking and it was lovely to see that dry theory working in practice as the group flourished and gained confidence. I hope that the Forget Me Not edition of Ramblings will help others realise that even with dementia you can still enjoy the outdoors, you can still get hot and sweaty, get lost, get wet in the rain and come out the other side of it a happier, healthier person.

Clare Balding, Ramblings, BBC Radio 4

The Forget Me Not Centre, based in Swindon, facilitates and supports its members as far as possible to reclaim, develop and maintain satisfying, productive and enjoyable lives, to live positively with dementia. This is based firmly on the philosophy that occupation and activity give meaning to life, promote health and well-being, and that health is strongly influenced by having choice and control in everyday occupation.

The Hiking Group meets weekly and together walks many miles of countryside. Everyone takes a part in the many roles and tasks needed to ensure the group is enjoyable, fulfilling, empowering and appropriately challenging, for all members.

The Swindon Hiking Group

Activities are important

Living with the effects of dementia can at times be frightening, frustrating and difficult. One day you may not be able to find your way around the supermarket, remember your pin number or give the right money on the bus. Maybe searching for the right words to express yourself or difficulty dealing with some paperwork has felt overwhelming. You may have had trouble with the remote control for the TV, with making a meal or remembering the detail of what your friend told you last time she was on the phone. All this might make you feel useless, low and frustrated.

These things may have been difficult for some time. Perhaps your illness has progressed, resulting in your husband or wife, family or friends assisting you to take care of things such as finances and admin, arranging appointments, cooking, driving, booking a holiday, sorting out repairs to the house, shopping or laundry.

Activities in which you can get really engaged and that give you an opportunity to accomplish something, particularly with others, may seem reduced. There may be fewer opportunities to do the things of your choice that are meaningful to you and provide a level of challenge that can test, but not overwhelm, and therefore offer a sense of achievement and success.

Activities that were previously taken for granted can now seem daunting, with the potential for frustration and embarrassment if they can't be carried out to previous standards.

Dementia, indeed any chronic and debilitating condition, may result in looking at life from a different perspective. Previously held values and beliefs about what is important in life may change. What seemed so important before – the deadline for a report at work, the tidying up, whether or not you've cleaned the car, your argument with your kids or spouse, where to go on holiday – may not seem so important now. You may now see life in a different light. Partners or friends may also experience a shift in their perspectives, and this may or may not be in line with yours. Everyone's emotional responses to the effects of a diagnosis of dementia are different, and coming to terms with the changes to life that happen as a result can be tough for many.

So what can help along this journey? There are some basic principles about the way we live, the things we do and what keeps us healthy and happy as human beings. The core philosophy of occupational therapy asserts that the occupations in which a person engages have an extremely powerful effect on their health and happiness.

We should aim to maintain and re-establish occupations and activities that are meaningful, that we have chosen, and provide an appropriate level of challenge to enable satisfaction and achievement.

These activities should include looking after ourselves and our homes, leisure and relaxation, and contributing to and engaging with our families and communities – having a role and feeling useful.

In short, all the activities we do in life help to meet our spiritual, mental, emotional and physical human needs. They support health, safety, relationships, self-esteem, achievement, personal growth, meaning to life and making a difference.

In practical terms this means such things as re-establishing an active and enjoyable social life, meeting others with similar problems and regaining self-confidence. It is often enabled by doing things we want to do, need to do and enjoy, re-establishing previous interests and beginning new ones, and continuing as far as we are able to actively participate in the running of our own life. It is important to feel that we have a useful role in life, are not afraid to make mistakes, have confidence that life can go on with dementia and learn to use alternative strategies and practical aids to manage memory problems. Often the way you experience illness, its symptoms and the course it takes are altered, depending on effective engagement in occupation.

Our experience of who we are is characterised by our memories and commitments of the past, the excitement of the present, and our dreams and hopes for the future.

As humans with or without dementia we actively engage in life, we strive to create meaning from everything we encounter and to understand the contradictions we face. We need to express who we are, to engage with the world and others at an emotional level and to share knowledge, ideas and creativity. Humans are at their happiest when they are busy, enjoying, overcoming, choosing, challenging, finding meaning, in flow and balance.

In the first instance most people turn to the doctor – to get an accurate diagnosis is important, but everyone's journey with this illness is different. How do you cope? What effects will the diagnosis have? How will it affect your relationships with others?

What affects you one day may not be the same tomorrow; dementia brings with it many challenges to everyday life.

Whilst there may be many effects on what you are able to do, being proactive about finding new, achievable and engaging ways of spending time is crucial. Many people have huge transitions in how they like to spend their time as they progress through the life cycle.

Of the many ways dementia can affect you, not all have to be seen in a negative light. Time spent trying new things can open doors and be transformational. Spending time outdoors in the countryside can provide experiences which lead to the acquisition and maintenance of new skills and competencies that can benefit many other aspects of life in your journey living with dementia.

Our Hiking Group

On Wednesdays we take to the hills (or fields, or forests, or mud, or moors...). Going out is what we do...

For our Hiking Group, preparation begins on Tuesday nights, when everyone gets an early night for the long Wednesday ahead and begins contemplating the weather and the snow, downpour or fog that tomorrow might bring. Different people wonder, 'Did I clean my boots from last week, where are my walking trousers, my bus pass, rucksack?' Talk begins the day before – who's in, where shall we go, any thoughts? Walking around the supermarket wondering what we can buy that everyone will like, or what would be a change. Don't spend too long; everyone will be waiting to get on. Walk in, familiar faces, dogs, bread-buttering and flask-filling, going to the loo.

Make it to the cars. Maps photocopied. Have we got everything? We have a vague agreement as to a plan. Lots to consider – whether we'll get lost, how cold and wet is it? Are we up for it? What happened last week? What's the general mood? Is it a day for a forest or a view for miles or a walk we know well, or a new one with lots of debate about the way?

So what's really going on? Getting out, fresh air. For centuries, probably since the beginning of time, people have wondered about nature, and our human need to be in it cannot be underestimated, especially when a disease comes along that can erode skills and our sense of self. What do we gather meaning from? How do we relate to others? What can we engage in and enjoy?

You don't have to talk to anyone, or if you are bored you can drop back and talk to someone else. There are no rules, it makes you feel young. It's being lost, being cold, being frustrated. It's not easy, but you don't get to see the amazing things we see in the countryside in the street! The countryside is astounding. You never know what you are going to see, and it enables people to chat. There's a mission, a goal, a sense of pleasure, something to talk about with others.

As Jim says:

> Sometimes I carry the lead (with or without a dog on it, depending on where we are!). I never mind carrying the rucksack – it means I've got the food! We encounter risk. We just passed a fairly deep stream that should have been the path. We built a walkway out of logs and branches as a team and we all got across safely. Everyone was a bit anxious, but drawing on past knowledge we helped each other, had to listen and be patient. All mucked in and did it.
>
> We walk, chat, and see things in different weathers, when it's flooded or dry, green, grey and wet, all white, frosty or muddy. It's different from week to week, surprises, all that snow, birds, flowers, plants, it's what enables you to relate to being alive and part of it all.
>
> So why get us (people living with dementia) together? Is it better that we all have dementia? Could we get the same benefit from meeting with a group of people without the illness? In this way, our world is equal, we meet and all is equal. It gives me a chance to achieve in a non-judgemental environment, don't have to look or feel like a fool, or put energy in trying to behave 'normally', because we are normal, we just want to carry on. Getting over problems like getting lost in the fog, or over a river, or a changed route because of an electric fence, a broken stile or a field of cows. Forgetting the picnic cups and asking the local country pub to lend us some for a few hours led to lots of laughter, sharing and a memorable pint! Challenges turn into the best adventures. It's all part of it. Interestingly, on Wednesdays I feel like I have a day away from Alzheimer's when I don't have to worry about it.

Furthermore, it's easy to live in a false, protected or limited world, but out in nature, whoever it's with, others with similar problems, friends, family or a local group, hiking in the countryside is levelling and something we can all enjoy together. Being outside offers a rich and fertile opportunity for conversation, gives something to remember, and gives something to learn. It helps to enable and empower people to reach their potential and live fulfilling lives.

Clare Balding from Radio 4 joined our Swindon-based Forget Me Not group of people with early-onset dementia for our walk through the Wiltshire countryside and discovered a very lively group who share a lot of laughs along the way (see below). The message we are keen to portray is that a diagnosis of dementia doesn't mean the end of a happy or fulfilling life. We get together once a week to walk for several hours and find that walking not only stimulates the mind, but helps us to overcome anxieties and problems to do with the loss of confidence and self-esteem that stems from having the disease.

A synopsis of the BBC Radio 4 programme 'Ramblings'
The conversations below describe what happens on one of our walks.[1]

> *Lynda*: 'Right, are we ready then? Have we all got a copy of the instructions? I haven't, so does anyone know where we are going?'
>
> [Laughter.] 'Yeah… We're walking down that way.' After a fair bit of discussion and debate, off we set…
>
> *Lynda*: The group are people who've all had a diagnosis of early-onset dementia (such as Alzheimer's, Lewy body or frontal lobe dementia). On the whole they're under 65.
>
> The point of the group? We come hiking, nobody is really in charge. We try to encourage people to come out, socialise, take some exercise, they join in shopping, making a picnic, deciding where we are going, following the instructions and basically to get people to carry on living as normal a life as possible. Really, we let them 'get on with it', so if we are going to get lost we're going to get lost! Come rain or shine we go. On the whole, the more difficult the day and the more inclement the weather, the more exciting it is and the more everyone remembers it, funnily enough!
>
> *Ian*: We walk between five and six miles, sometimes more and sometimes less – you can never really trust guided walks but on the whole we're out for about four to five hours. It's an overcast day but warm, only a marginal threat of rain, the group is about 14 with lots of kit. We've got heated water for tea and coffee, we've got loads of food, we've always got too much food, in fact I reckon I've put

---

1   Available at www.bbc.co.uk/programmes/b00tw5xt, broadcast on 25 September 2010.

on weight since I started in November last year and it's been great. It's fabulous because, you know, I was running a dental surgery for 30–35 years, and suddenly it all stopped. Although my wife and I have done a bit of travelling, this gets me out and also gives my wife a break. It's great, they're very interesting people and the girls who organise it are great. If we went straight on at the bottom of the hill, we'd come eventually to Jamie's land, that's Jamie down there, the tallest guy, he's got a farm over there, it's no distance from my town but I've never walked here until now! Amazing really, just your local stuff, on your doorstep, it's great, let's hop over this stile.

Going over the stile, Elaine's dementia at times gives her trouble with body perception – sometimes she's not sure where she's putting her feet down and we all offer her a bit of help. We all help each other and I think she secretly loves being carried over by all us strong men!

I think my memory was affected way before I ever had this, it was my wife, my best friend, my [dental] hygienist who's worked with me for 21 years, and friends who began to think things were going a bit pear-shaped.

I was really having trouble driving, which was the other thing that started to make life difficult for me. I just wasn't putting the car in the place it should be. I was doing a clinic at the hospital every week, but actually every time I parked the car I'd look at it and think that I hadn't parked very well and I'd go back to the car and change/improve it. Did it frighten me? No not really, well, I was frightened driving and then quite relieved to be not involved with driving anymore. It took us over a year to get a diagnosis; I think it was as difficult for my wife as it was for me. I stopped work, and had to just get on with it, you know. That's the other thing about this, we come out and have a laugh and we do have a lot…a lot…of fun, and even when we get lost we are enriched by the adventure of it… Ahh, there's the high-speed train between London and Wales whizzing by…

Clare [chats to the microphone informing her Radio 4 listeners]: The centre itself, I ought to explain, is based in Swindon, and the group met there at ten o' clock in the morning, and it's now half past twelve, and we've got another, yep, we've got more stiles to get over. So it's a very, very easy, relaxed social beginning, no pressure of time and everybody allowed to find their own rhythm. And that is vital.

Derek [reads out loud from the guide book]: Continue across another two stiles and down the track beyond in the same direction, keeping parallel with the railway.

Clare: Now, Derek, how come you can read that out and it sounds totally straightforward?

Derek: 'Cause I'm a man, ahh no, oh no, no, if my daughters hear that they'll kill me! No, it's because of my technical background. I can read it and make it sound straightforward. And it makes me read out loud, I get to practise – some people find reading hard, practice can help.

Clare: What did you do, what's your job?

Derek: I joined the air force at 16 and did three years' training in aircraft electronics and then carried on with that until I left the air force when I was 35. From there I went into childcare, which was totally different, and then reverted to be a technical trainee.

Clare: And when did you stop working?

Derek: When I finally retired I got involved in setting up a wood recycling company, and that was about five years ago, and then two years into that was when the Alzheimer's started to appear. I really thought I couldn't be a director of a company, it sounded great – 'I'm a director of a company.'

Clare: And how did the Alzheimer's manifest itself?

Derek: I started to realise that a) I was forgetting things, and b) I was struggling if I was trying to do a calculation in my head, and if somebody buys 20 metres of wood at 25p a metre I used to be able to calculate it immediately. I also noticed that when somebody would come into the wood yard for something, I wouldn't remember that they'd been in the week before and bought 20 quid's worth of wood, I'd start to show them round, and they'd be like, yeah, you did this last week, and that sort of brought it home to me as well.

Clare: And how do you find the walking helps?

Derek: Well, I think it's my third walk, there's a bunch of people who are very relaxed and don't seem to worry about Alzheimer's, we all pull together, I get some confidence back. I learn patience and understanding too. Also, l think I'm not very much a burden on my wife at the moment, and this helps it to stay that way. It keeps me active, fit, my mind engaged, and you've got demands made of you, just enough to make you feel challenged and a bit uncomfortable and great when you manage it, whether it's making the tea for everyone (which is no mean feat), climbing a steep hill or helping someone who's having a bit of trouble. Like I say, it helps me be confident at home and carry on having a go at things. A bad day today doesn't mean a bad day tomorrow. Oh, and the time may come when she'll be only too pleased for me to come out for a day walking and give her a bit of peace, knowing that I'm safe and doing something I love.

Clare: It's interesting that Ian said that as well, it gives his wife a real break.

Derek: Yeah, and I do feel that, I'm going to be preaching here, you should never take things away from people that they can do. Also it boosts me up when I'm doing things. When I finished this and think 'Ooh, I've done that,' you feel such a sense of normality.

Clare: Do you find that one of the side effects is that confidence has been shot to pieces because you don't trust yourself anymore, and that other people don't trust you either to do the things you used to be able to do?

Derek: Yeah, in the past if something went wrong, you'd stop and work out what was going wrong. But now the confidence goes and you think, 'Well it's not necessary,' something's gone wrong outside of you, as it probably was in the past, but you immediately think, 'Oh no, what I have I done now?' I know I've messed something up, and it sort of puts me back a bit, but then you go and do something good for a bit and you think, 'That last one was a glitch, this is what I really do.' Yeah, and if you can't manage to do it the one day it doesn't mean you can't manage the next day. Yeah, you do have different days.

Clare [to Lynda]: So tell us some more about the Forget Me Not Centre and your role?

Lynda: I'm an occupational therapist. In the UK there are limited services for people with early-onset dementia and your needs are so different if you get it young. So I think if people could feel more relaxed about it, can feel it's not the end of the world and you can go on living, it is of enormous benefit. Early diagnosis can really help because understanding and accepting what you've got is the very start of being able to deal with it. If you don't know what it is and you are living in fear – that's paralysing and debilitating. Without diagnosis and support to accept it and find new ways of living, a person's social network can disintegrate and careers can end in trauma due to poor performance rather than ill health. Talking to family and friends about it can make an enormous difference

Listen, from the other side of the hedge that ripple of laughter – everybody is relaxed and enjoying themselves. It's very uncompetitive. It's not about who knows the way and who doesn't.

One of the effects of having Alzheimer's, as with many illnesses, is that you're looked after, so you can lose the chance to be useful to other people. All of us need to be useful to others and have meaningful roles to feel good about our own existence. With this group of people they all help each other out, everybody experiences problems in different ways, helping and needing are swapped and reciprocated throughout the day. It's a beautiful group to be with. Sometimes Elaine can get over the stiles and it's no problem. Other times she's not sure where her feet and legs are, and different people help her in different ways at different times. It's such an unpredictable illness, it affects everybody differently, so there is no set path or timescale. We have clients who remain stable for long periods and others have very rapid changes. When anybody gets diagnosed, the message in the media is so often the end stage and people forget there are thousands of people at earlier stages striving to live 'normal' and fulfilling lives with just a bit of support when it's needed. Most people don't die of Alzheimer's, they die of other things along the way and can carry on having a fulfilled and enjoyable life if you're not too scared to keep on living.

Clare: Hi, Sandy, someone told me you've got great tips for remembering things.

Sandy: I'm excellent! I'm not really, and names are my worst. I can't remember names, my granddaughter! I couldn't remember and Lynda came up with this thing. Sherry's quite warm, not the song 'Sherry' but sherry the drink, and nine times out of ten I remember it. You know, our Natasha, she has a moustache she hates us for remembering her name like that – Tasha.

Clare: The last 40 minutes of the walk were spent stuck in a field that we shouldn't have been in, not knowing the way out.

Conclusion

We are all engaged and fulfilled in life by what we do and by making the most of the opportunities life offers. To walk on a Wednesday involves a weekly commitment, preparation days before, weariness for some time after, and ongoing laughter and pleasure at what we remember.

Our weekly countryside walk is a vehicle for interaction, communication and building confidence, and for maintaining and growing skills that transfer to everyday life. With every walk clients build and grow their armoury for dealing with an ever-changing life context and face it with renewed confidence, re-energised by a Wednesday success. The fact that a PIN number was forgotten on Tuesday and a mobile phone call was impossible on Sunday pales into insignificance after a triumphant walk on Wednesday. The challenges and joys we share as we walk help not only to put the daily struggles we face into perspective, but also to rejuvenate us and give us renewed confidence to continue to try and live the best life we can.

Chapter 5

From Demedicalisation to Renaturalisation

Dementia and Nature in Harmony

PETER WHITEHOUSE, DANNY GEORGE,
JOHANNA WIGG AND BRETT JOSEPH

The enormity of the challenges of dementia for individuals, families, communities and the world as a whole requires our deepest collective wisdom. We need to engage our whole selves – mind, body and spirit – in summoning meaningful human responses to these daunting challenges, and we need to develop a clear sense of priorities accompanied by a healthy scepticism about medical and technologically-based promises of an ultimate solution to brain ageing. Yet, intrinsic to the notion of wisdom is recognition of limits – the limits of our own human abilities to frame and solve problems, as well as the limits of the bounties that nature offers to responsible stewards. Just as dementia is defined by cognitive impairment sufficient to impair activities of daily living, our species is beginning to become imbued with the wisdom of knowing that our accustomed patterns of unlimited consumption and waste generation are dramatically impairing the functioning of ecosystems that sustain our collective presence on the planet.

The journey towards the future must be to promote social engagement of elders and the health of communities in general. We must confront dogmatic positivism (excessive faith in science and technology) and confront excessive medicalisation in the way we conceptualise dementia-related challenges. Scientists are constantly in danger of losing their humility by professing to know more than they know. The echoes of the optimism for brain psychiatry as practised by Alois Alzheimer over 100 years ago still resonate in our universities and drug companies today. Ironically, the imaginations of our scientists can be dulled by the seductive power of image-rich technologies, whether involving a cell stain creating a rich microscopic image in 1910 or a PET scan doing so today.

These technologies, while offering new ways to visualise complex brain functions, tend to draw attention away from the basic tasks of human adaptation, whereby words and stories matter as much as neurons and brains in the project of improving the quality of life; for those with dementia and, in fact, for all of us. We must renaturalise persons with dementia and ourselves by embracing the intimate and healing relationships that emerge when we live with nature instead of trying to control it.

Our use of the word 'renaturalise,' which is a modification of the more familiar word 'naturalise,' is deliberate. The latter word has been assigned multiple definitions, including the following:

> 1: to confer the rights of a national on; *especially*: to admit to citizenship, 2: to introduce into common usage or into the vernacular, 3: to bring into conformity with nature, [and] 4: to cause (as a plant) to become established as if native. (Merriam-Webster 2011)

We see our coinage of the word '*re*naturalise' as a useful and appropriate way of connoting the process of re-establishing a relationship that once existed and of inviting a deeper inquiry into overlapping meanings.

Specifically, it is a call to bring people with dementia into full citizenship of their communities, both through socialisation with other human beings and by building ever-deepening connection with the larger community of life and the Earth itself. We also claim that we could all benefit from that quest. Later, we use the term 'postmodern' in referring to the present cultural context of our challenges with dementia, largely to signify that there are massive changes still underway in society, of a nature and scale that portend the end of one era and the beginning of another.

Healing power of nature

The power of nature to heal is well recognised in many indigenous cultures and in so-called complementary and alternative medicine. In contrast, Western allopathic medicine tends to see nature as inimical, with the human intellect combating the alien invasion by disease of the human body and mind. Power is seen as residing in the doctor as expert. Little role is assigned to the person with the condition, who rather is directed to play the role of a passive recipient of the ministrations of the physician. Also, to the extent that healing approaches utilising art and caring can be associated with even Western scientific medicine, such approaches are often neglected (e.g. humanistic approaches are under-reimbursed by health insurances and health services of various kinds) when compared with the seduction of powerful and expensive invasive procedures.

Today, however, we are living through a time of rapid changes in society, the environment, and technology, with far-reaching cultural implications. We believe rethinking and revaluing dementia can be a part of that larger cultural transformation. The areas of health ecology, horticultural therapy, and healing landscapes are increasingly being recognized as legitimate areas of health science and practice (Honari and Boleyn 1999). Evidence is accumulating for specific approaches, particularly those focusing on attentional mechanisms and relaxation, and are proving effective in specific conditions (Devlin and Arneil 2003; Sternberg 2009). Moreover, architectural design and now landscape design are being increasingly applied in health organisational planning. Designing physical spaces that are dementia-friendly is a particular imperative and challenge, given the variability in the pattern of and degrees of cognitive difficulties. Learning environments for children and adults are receiving more design attention. Finally, the green building movement is influencing many new building projects as we work towards reducing the ecological footprint of our built environment.

In this chapter, we illustrate ways of living in greater harmony with ourselves and of keeping life-long learning and environmental stewardship at the heart of our communities. We will see the value both for those with ageing-associated cognitive challenges and for all of us. We use the power of both qualitative and quantitative approaches, narrative and data, to create our picture of the need for change.

The Vicarage by the Sea

The mission of The Vicarage by the Sea is to develop a setting within which individuals living with progressive, neurologically debilitating diseases can live, grow and flourish with peers, family and staff. Intrinsic to the creation of this setting is the presence of the natural world, including pets, such as dogs and cats. In addition, residents have full access to the outdoors. They may engage with nature as they see fit and when they choose. The Vicarage mission recognises the human need and desire, regardless of age or ailment, for connection with the beauty of nature and its healing properties.

In the mid-1990s, American models for long-term dementia care were largely institutional, with locked doors, and little if any contact with the natural world. Founded in 1998, The Vicarage introduced many distinguishing features, including nurturing residents' engagement with the natural world. The Vicarage is located in a rural, wooded landscape (Figure 5.1), overlooking the Atlantic Ocean. There are beautiful flower gardens and plenty of wildlife to watch.

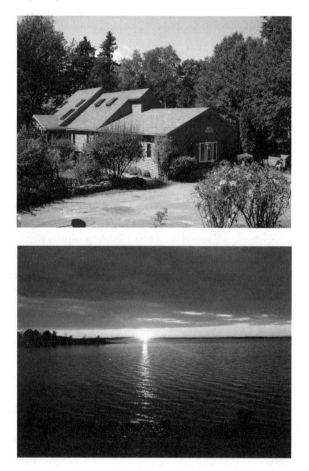

Figure 5.1 The Vicarage by the Sea
Photos: Cheryl Golek

During the first few years of operation, many residents moved into The Vicarage with pets, creating a rich environment for all. Moving from a home setting into an institutional setting is traumatic (Danermark and Ekstrom 1990; Fisher 1990). Being forced to leave a beloved pet further traumatises elders confused by relocation. The Vicarage philosophically commits to the psychological and social well-being of its residents by honouring the healing/comforting effects of connecting with the natural world. While relocation for individuals living with dementia is challenging and stressful (Lander, Brazill and Landrigan 1997; Robertson, Warrington and Eagles 1993), the residents' stress and anxiety are lessened by having a pet nearby for comfort (Figure 5.2).

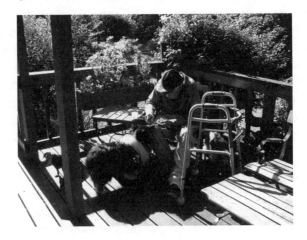

Figure 5.2 A resident of The Vicarage with his pet dog
Photo: Cheryl Golek

> Veronica moved to The Vicarage with her loyal yellow lab, Ginny. Ginny followed her owner everywhere. When Veronica went outdoors for a walk, her dog followed. Ginny was her companion in all settings and moods. As Veronica's anxiety rose, Ginny stayed close providing unconditional attention and love. After a walk and some petting of her dog, Veronica's demeanour visibly relaxed.

> Alice moved in with her corgi, Harry. While the dog monitored the running of the home, Alice oversaw her loyal friend. She displayed obvious satisfaction in keeping track of her dog and his needs. If the dog barked, she apologised for his behaviour, displaying purposefulness in pet ownership.

Flora moved to The Vicarage with two dachshunds, Myrna and Leanne. The dogs were like Flora's children. She coddled them when she was stressed, ran with them outdoors when she was happy, and simply loved them. Her dogs offered Flora a mothering role that visibly satisfied her sense of identity.

Incorporation of residents' pets builds on The Vicarage's mission of sustaining a setting that encourages residents' growth.

Another distinguishing feature of The Vicarage model is its commitment to a secure facility without locked doors. The Vicarage uses simple technology to monitor the whereabouts of its residents. The Vicarage's philosophy honours residents' needs to enter the outdoors. Many long-term dementia care settings require locked doors on the unit, arguing that locks provide safety for the residents (Coleman 1993; Noyes and Sliva 1993; Robinson *et al.* 2007). Locked doors often elevate anxiety for residents desiring to exit the premises. At The Vicarage, motion detectors alert staff to a resident's desire to go outdoors. The staffing ratio of one staff person to four residents permits staff to join the resident for a walk outside. In keeping with The Vicarage mission, residents determine when they would like to engage with nature.

Arthur spent his entire life fishing the ocean for lobsters. He was intimately connected to the sea and all its wonders. During the afternoon, when his anxiety rose, he wanted nothing more than to walk along the oceanside and search for creatures in the sand. While walking with staff, he pointed out clam air holes and crabs hiding under seaweed. The simple process of walking in a natural environment reduced his anxiety and cleared his mind.

Patricia gardened her entire life and loved nothing more than to meander onto the deck and prune the many plants and flowers adorning the railing. She lived with anxiety which peaked at various times of the day. When she became anxious, she simply walked onto the deck and focused on the beauty of nature. The reduction in stress and anxiety visibly diminished while she tended to the flowers.

Harold was drawn to sunlight as if it were a drug. In the morning, he watched the sunrise to see whether there would be sunshine or not. In the event that the sun appeared, he gathered his coat and entered the outdoors for a nice walk. A member of staff joined him and Harold shared memories of times he spent in the wilderness.

> He was a keen observer of wildlife and enjoyed watching the turkeys
> roam the property. After a walk, Harold relaxed and read the paper,
> visibly content.

Some residents wish to sit outside in the sunshine, while others enjoy a walk up the country lane or down to the oceanside. For many residents, simply being able to breathe fresh air calms their anxiety and relaxes their feelings. The incorporation of both animals and access to the natural world emphasises The Vicarage's commitment to challenging the medical model of long-term dementia care. By creating a care setting that reaps the benefits of nature, anxiety levels diminish and reliance on pharmacological support is lessened.

After 13 years, The Vicarage's mission continues to redefine long-term dementia care. The incorporation of the natural world helps to demedicalise the lives of its residents, and nurture amongst them a shared sense of being in relationship with their fellow human beings and with the other sentient beings that populate their natural surroundings. The Vicarage's 'culture of dementia' (Wigg 2007) emphasises its residents' citizenship (Bartlett and O'Connor 2007) through its focus on residents' needs and abilities, rather than their diseases. At The Vicarage, renaturalisation occurs among peers living with progressive neurological diseases who choose to engage with one another and their natural world. In this way, The Vicarage aims to transform a preoccupation with deficit into the personally rewarding experience of being meaningfully engaged as a participant within a perpetually-renewing community of life.

The Intergenerational School

The mission of The Intergenerational School (TIS) is to create an educational community of excellence where learners from kindergarten through elderhood develop the skills and experiences necessary for life-long learning and spirited citizenship. The curriculum is developmentally-based and includes older people (and younger) in cognitive challenges. Hence, children work and learn with people with dementia who both come to the school to read to children and allow youngsters to visit them in their long-term care communities (Figure 5.3).

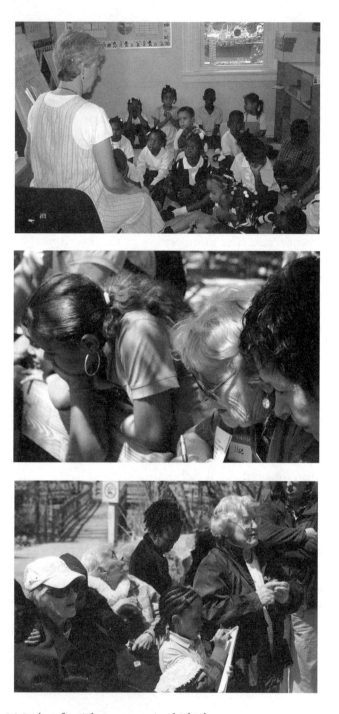

Figure 5.3 Students from The Intergenerational School
Photos: Peter Whitehouse

Since its inception in 2000, TIS has become a high-performing K-8 charter school[1] that serves 224 inner-city students in multi-age classrooms and is structured around the ideology that people of all ages can learn alongside each other throughout their lifespan. Students are placed in multi-age classrooms, based on individual learning needs, where they learn in their own way and at their own pace, moving along five developmental stages and advancing to the next learning stage once they demonstrate mastery of the stage benchmarks. The school's founders, the first author of this chapter (Peter Whitehouse, a geriatric neurologist) and his wife Catherine (a child psychologist), shared a conviction that educational environments should not be institutions of age-segregation, but places of age-integration where rich lessons from our elders' past combine with youthful imaginings about the future. They believed that the process of learning was not categorically different for children and adults, and that schools could be places where people of all ages learn alongside one another.

The school has been rated 'Excellent' by the Ohio Department of Education, based on standardised test scores for six out of the seven years it was eligible to be assessed. It has received local, regional, national, and international recognition and awards as a high-performing urban school providing high-quality learning experiences for children. We have also found that participation in intergenerational volunteering at the school reduces stress for people with mild to moderate dementia (George and Singer 2010; George and Whitehouse 2010).

Having established that TIS measurably benefits younger and older learners, we have sought to build on previous work (see Stenig and Butts 2010) in designing collaborative programmes that foster intergenerational dialogue and action around some of the most urgent issues of our era (Ingman, Benjamin, and Lusky 1999). Beginning in 2010, TIS launched an intergenerational nature programme with our local nature centre. The Nature Centre at Shaker Lakes programme aspires to bring the generations together through experiential, intergenerational learning in the parklands and watersheds that surround TIS, with the ultimate goal of nurturing a sense of place, fostering a deeper understanding of systems-based thinking in nature, and building reverence – what the naturalist Rachel Carson called 'a sense of wonder' – for the natural world (Carson

---

1   A K-8 charter means an elementary school (ages 5 to 14) which is a public (i.e. government-funded) but not a regular school system school, so that it is more independent and free to be innovative.

1965). For the past three semesters, students have joined elders from a local assisted-living facility on several visits to a local nature centre where they have learned about such topics as habitats, wetland ecology, weather concepts and observations, water quality, chemical testing, macro-invertebrate sampling, wetlands, woods and soil testing (Figure 5.4).

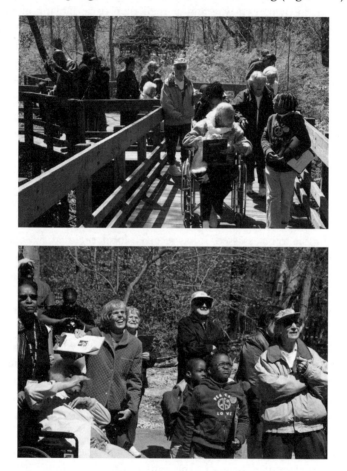

Figure 5.4 The Intergenerational School's nature programme
Photos: Danny George (top) and Peter Whitehouse (bottom)

Students partner with elders on experiential exercises that help them learn the art of scientific inquiry and to acquire the vocabulary needed to build a conceptual foundation about responsibilities for being stewards of nature. During each visit, elders assist students in framing questions about environmental concepts, conducting deep observations in cohorts, writing (and drawing) reflectively, and identifying interrelationships and patterns, drawing conclusions to questions posed by nature centre educators, and producing collaborative pieces of artwork or other reflective projects that convey what was learned.

At the time of writing, information technology experts from Case Western Reserve University are helping develop a social media platform that will enable online exchange between elders and students on topical issues in the nature-based curriculum. Text, pictures and video can be shared through this platform, thus extending and enriching the conversation beyond the hands-on experience. An augmented environment will also be created, using the social networking application Second Life to allow students and elders to work together to model their local environment and visualise it from a virtual perspective that overlays their real-life experience. This will provide a new online platform within which narrative exchange and action regarding complex environmental systems can occur.

Through these visits, we learned that several elder participants were members of a grassroots advocacy group called the 'Freeway Fighters' that had successfully lobbied to save the host nature centre from being developed into a superhighway in the 1960s. Exchange of intergenerational narrative with older people who have lived the history of the nature centre has grounded experiential learning in the moment, while also nurturing a long-term perspective within a larger historical context that imbues the intergenerational, nature-based activity with greater meaning and relevance for younger students. Creating shared spaces where older people (some of whom are affected by dementia) can educate younger children about a significant aspect of their life story fosters opportunities for increased sense of purpose and the furthering of a legacy.

Dementia and wisdom for a sustainable world

In the preceding examples, we described two current contexts in which the challenges of dementia are met with creative and adaptive responses that challenge the prevailing medical model, with the intention of counteracting its dehumanising aspects. By pursuing an agenda of renaturalising dementia from an experiential, social and environmental perspective, these innovators demonstrate how refocusing interventions away from a myopic pre-occupation with technology-driven cures, towards a holistic, quality-of-life orientation encompassed within the idea of natural citizenship, improves the prospects for healthy adaptation within a world bounded by natural limits.

As we proceed along life's journey in the context of a changing (some say postmodern) world, those of us who face the prospect of cognitive impairment will gain little comfort from promises of ultimate cures that reflect the positivist orientation of our current technologically and scientifically-driven culture. The predominantly mechanistic worldview that shaped the daily realities of the passing industrial era is giving way to an information-driven world that challenges our human capacity for adaptation in the face of rapid change. In the absence of a predominant guiding story to replace the yesterday's themes of 'progress' and 'manifest destiny,' we citizens of the twenty-first century in a post-industrial age stand to face a crisis of meaning that is amplified by a profound sense of alienation from the natural world that is our culture's legacy.

In a spiritless, mechanised world, cognition becomes the cornerstone of all that we define as our humanity. However, as our Western society comes of age within an information-rich and culturally diverse cultural context, aspects of our human potential that have been long overlooked are now coming to light. From this perspective, our generation's struggle to come to terms with dementia may best be understood within the context of the larger cultural transformation that is implied by the current popular interest in sustainability and associated concepts. Engaging people with cognitive impairment in a culture of dementia as citizens, be it in a home residence or a school, is part of this transformation. This diffusion of transformative thought and action under the banner of sustainability is informed by converging threads of inquiry (e.g. in the areas of human science, eco-psychology, humanistic and existential psychology, integral studies, systems theory, mind–body medicine, appreciative inquiry, indigenous spirituality, applied and activist social science and eco-feminism).

A guiding premise linking these diverse pathways of inquiry is the notion that the value and quality of human life as inherited via the modern worldview, severely underestimates human potential and overlooks those participatory dimensions of our existence that, when validated and shared within a given cultural context, can open human consciousness to profound and meaningful experiences aligned with Nature's own wisdom.

Such wisdom stresses the importance of communities of living creatures supporting each other, and for human beings to develop a sense of stewardship with a long-term perspective. The Vicarage by the Sea and The Intergenerational School illustrate this kind of life-affirming and life-spanning community. They recognise the importance of emotions as well as cognition in motivating us to procreate and protect our young as our future selves, and our elders as rich sources of knowledge of the past.

Dementia should teach us all humility. We are all at risk of brain damage due to a variety of causes, from head injuries and toxic exposures to age-related processes. More profoundly, our environmental challenges should show us all that we are impaired in our own activities of daily living as a species. We do not produce and consume food using healthy processes, and we discharge our 'waste' in ways that damage our own home, Planet Earth.

One of us (Peter Whitehouse) had the pleasure and honour of meeting Arne Naess, the Norwegian philosopher, mountaineer, and environmental activist who invented the concept of 'deep ecology' (see Chapter 14 in this book). His ideas emphasised the importance of appreciating the depths of our connectedness to nature, not just in biological but also in cultural and spiritual ways. He popularised the metaphor that human beings need to 'think like a mountain' i.e. long-term, broad-based, with lofty aspirations. Even as he developed dementia himself, Arne inspired the whole nation of Norway and beyond to take their stewardship responsibilities seriously, but with a playful attitude about life.

Conclusion

Although we cannot assume that any particular individual who jumps on the sustainability bandwagon is necessarily motivated by an interest in changing worldviews or cultural transformation, as Arne Naess was, those of us who face the challenge of dementia may well discover that our greatest nemesis is not the fact of cognitive impairment, but the cultural burden that prevents us from experiencing dementia, not as dreaded loss of identity and meaning as implied by the predominant medical model with its zero-sum focus on cognitive impairments, but as a potentially emancipatory unfolding of previously hidden human potentials – including potentials invoked by the experience of deep interpersonal and transpersonal connectedness – the wholeness of the self-in-relationship

Our call to 'renaturalise' in response to the challenge of dementia may be understood as a call to re-imagine and revise our relationship with the myriad beings that constitute the life world. By re-engaging as sentient, embodied beings within the participatory and inter-subjective world of nature, we honour the delimited patterns and cycles of the natural world in ways that invite a transformed understanding of the value and quality of human life. In other words, it is only by accepting Mother Nature's embrace that we may realise the true meaning of human emancipation.

References

Bartlett, R. and O'Connor, D. (2007) 'From personhood to citizenship: Broadening the lens for dementia practice and research.' *Journal of Aging Studies 21*, 107–118.

Carson, R. (1965) *The Sense of Wonder*. New York: Harper and Row.

Coleman, E.A. (1993) 'Physical restraint use in nursing home patients with dementia.' *Journal of the American Medical Association 270*, 17, 2114–2115.

Danermark, B. and Ekstrom, M. (1990) 'Relocation and health effects on the elderly: A commented research review.' *Journal of Sociology and Social Welfare 25*, 25–49.

Devlin, A.S. and Arneil, A.B. (2003) 'Healthcare environments and patient outcomes: A review of the literature.' *Environment and Behavior 35*, 665–694.

Fisher, B. (1990) 'The stigma of relocation to a retirement facility.' *Journal of Aging Studies 4*, 47–59.

George, D.R. and Singer, M. (2010) 'Intergenerational volunteering and quality of life for persons with mild to moderate dementia: Results from a 5-month intervention study in the United States.' *American Journal of Geriatric Psychiatry 19*, 4, 249–396.

George, D.R. and Whitehouse, P.J. (2010) 'Can intergenerational volunteering enhance quality of life for persons with mild to moderate dementia? Results from a 5-month mixed methods intervention study in the United States.' *Journal of the American Geriatrics Society 58*, 4, 796–797.

Honari M. and Boleyn, T. (eds) (1999) *Health Ecology: Health, Culture and Human–Environment Interaction*. Routledge: London.

Ingman, S., Benjamin, T. and Lusky, R. (1999) 'The environment: The quintessential intergenerational challenge.' *Generations 22*, 4, 68–71.

Lander, S.M., Brazill, A.L. and Landrigan, P.M. (1997) 'Intra-institutional relocation: Effects on residents' behavior and psychosocial functioning.' *Journal of Gerontological Nursing 23*, 4, 35–41.

Merriam-Webster Dictionary online: 'Naturalize', accessed 25 February 2011 at www.merriam-webster.com/dictionary/naturalize.

Noyes, L.E. and Silva, M.C. (1993) 'The ethics of locked special care units for persons with Alzheimer's disease.' *American Journal of Alzheimer's Disease and Other Dementias 8*, 4, 12–15.

Robertson, C., Warrington, J. and Eagles, J.M. (1993) 'Relocation mortality in dementia: The effects of a new hospital.' *International Journal of Geriatric Psychiatry 8*, 521–525.

Robinson, L., Hutchings, D., Corner, L., Finch, T. *et al.* (2007) 'Balancing rights and risks: Conflicting perspectives in the management of wandering in dementia.' *Health, Risk, and Society 9*, 4, 389–406.

Stenig, S. and Butts, D. (2010) 'Generations going green: Intergenerational programs connecting young and old to improve our environment.' *Generations 33*, 64–69.

Sternberg, E.M. (2009) *Healing and Spaces: The Science of Place and Well-Being*. Cambridge, MA: Belknap Press.

Wigg, J.M. (2007) *A Culture of Dementia: Examining Interpersonal Relationships between Elders with Dementia*. PhD thesis, Brandeis University.

Further reading

Laszlo, C. (2010) 'Sustainable value in the pharmaceutical industry.' In *The Encyclopedia of Sustainability,* Vol. II. Gt Barrington, MA: Berkshire Publishing.

Marcus, C.B. and Barnes, M. (1999) *Healing Gardens: Therapeutic Benefits.* New York: John Wiley.

Potter, V.R. and Whitehouse, P.J. (1998) 'Deep and global bioethics for a livable third millennium.' *The Scientist 12,* 1, 9.

Ulrich, R.S. (1984) 'View through a window may influence recovery from surgery.' *Science 224,* 420–421.

Ulrich, R.S., Zimring, C.M., Zhu, X., DuBose, J. *et al.* (2008) 'A review of the research literature on evidence-based healthcare design.' *Health Environments Research and Design 1,* 3, 61–125.

Whitehouse, P.J. (2003) 'The rebirth of bioethics: extending the original formulations of Van Rensselaer Potter.' *American Journal of Bioethics 3,* 4, W26–W31.

Whitehouse, P.J. (2008) *The Myth of Alzheimer's: What You Aren't Being Told About Today's Most Dreaded Diagnosis.* New York: St. Martin's Griffin.

Whitehouse, P.J. and George, D. (2010a) 'Health – Public and Environmental.' In *The Encyclopedia of Sustainability,* Vol. II. Gt Barrington, MA: Berkshire Publishing.

Whitehouse, P.J. and George, D. (2010b) 'The Business of Sustainability.' In *The Encyclopedia of Sustainability,* Vol. II. Gt Barrington, MA: Berkshire Publishing.

Whitehouse, P.J. and George, D. (2010c) 'The Aesthetics of Natural Elderhood.' *Journal of Aging, Humanities, and the Arts 4,* 292–301.

A Walking Panacea

BRIAN AND JUNE HENNELL

There was a time many years ago
when things were bright, all systems go.
We laughed 'til we cried, no room for a sigh
'cept over some beauteous lullaby.

The mountains sang, church bells rang
to welcome each glorious day.
'Til I suddenly found that I'd lost my ground.
My framework was in disarray.

'You've dementia,' they said. 'Is that to do with my head?
Why are these things happening to me?'
This endless veil of uncertainty
cloaks me in misery.

Medication arrived and soon I worried
just how much of a change there would be?
But my dog was still there and surely he'll need to share
daily walks in the country with me?

I reach out and touch, Jack responds so much,
still there despite my recalcitrant mood.
Can this nightmare end now I've realised my friend
is ready our jaunts to renew?

The bulrushes dance and I am entranced
by the trees and canal-side scene.
Birds swooping in flight and other beautiful sights
keep my mood from being so mean.

I'm no longer stressed, my head not so messed
up with confusion and ready to fight.
This countryside ramble is the perfect preamble
for calmness which feels perfectly right.

When buds break forth each new Spring's dawn
and birds awake to charm each morn
I celebrate with unreserved cheer –
dementia or not, I'm still here.

For years and years I intend to be
healthily free, no risk assessment for me.
Each fresh air walk centres my life
into calmness and joy, with the help of my wife.

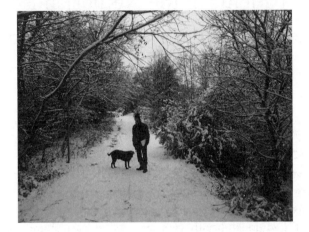

Brian Hennell with labrador Jack

Chapter 6

Farming for Health

Exploring the Benefits of Green Care Farms for Dementia Patients in the Netherlands

SIMONE DE BRUIN, SIMON OOSTING, MARIE-JOSÉ
ENDERS-SLEGERS AND JOS SCHOLS

Introduction

'Green care' is an umbrella term for a broad spectrum of health-promoting interventions, embracing living organisms (e.g. animals and plants) and natural elements (e.g. the weather). Green care links aspects of traditional health care systems to agriculture (green care farming), gardening (horticultural therapy), and animals (animal-assisted interventions). Green care creates a link between sectors that were formerly not linked, and may therefore create new benefits for all sectors involved (Haubenhofer, Elings, Hassink and Hine 2010; Hine, Peacock and Pretty 2008; Working Group on the Health Benefits of Green Care, COST 866 2010). In this chapter we focus on green care farming.

Green care farming relates to the use of commercial farms and agricultural landscapes as a base for promoting mental and physical health, through normal farming activity (Haubenhofer 2010; Hine 2008). All green care farms have some degree of 'farming' (i.e. crops, livestock, woodland) and of 'care' (i.e. health care, social rehabilitation, education, work training), but the ratio between farming and care, the type of farm (e.g. dairy farm, industrial livestock farm, mixed farm), and client groups all differ (Hassink 2007; Hine 2008). Main client groups of green care farms used to be people with a learning disability and patients with mental health problems. Since the beginning of the new millennium, however, green care farms have been providing health, social or educational services through farming for a wide range of people, including older people (with dementia), autistic children, people with burn-out, and long-term unemployed (Elings and Hassink 2006; Hassink *et al.* 2007; Hine *et al.* 2008).

Green care farming is developing in an increasing number of European countries, including the Netherlands, Norway, Belgium, Germany, Italy, Austria, Switzerland, and the United Kingdom (Hassink and Van Dijk 2006). There is much variety in green care farms over the different European countries. In the Netherlands, Norway, and Belgium, for example, green care farms are mostly private family farms, whereas in Germany and Austria green care farms are run by health care institutions. In Italy green care farms are social cooperatives (Haubenhofer *et al.* 2010). The number of green care farms differs considerably among countries. Currently the Netherlands is leading, with approximately 1000. Belgium, Norway, and Italy all have a few hundred green care farms, whereas in the UK, Finland, Sweden and Slovenia green care farming is a more recently established development. In these countries the number is limited to several dozen (Hassink and Van Dijk 2006).

This chapter gives insight into green care farming for people with dementia in the Netherlands and its effects on health outcomes of this client group.

Green care farming for dementia patients in the Netherlands

Green care farms for people with dementia mainly offer day care to this client group (De Bruin *et al.* 2009). A small number additionally offer small-scale living arrangements. We propose to focus on green care farms that offer day care (Roest *et al.* 2010). Day care facilities such as green care farms aim to develop a structured and meaningful day programme for people with dementia who live in the community. They additionally offer respite care to family caregivers by taking care of their relatives with dementia for an average of two or three days a week (Cohen-Mansfield *et al.* 2001; De Bruin *et al.* 2009, 2010b; Droës *et al.* 2004; Jarrott *et al.* 1998).

Green care farms are a valuable addition to the present care services for people with dementia living in the community and their family caregivers. With day care at green care farms the number of community services for people with dementia and their family caregivers has increased. Hence, people with dementia and their family caregivers may have more opportunities to find a service that best suits their preferences and interests. Services provided at green care farms are currently financed by the Dutch national insurance system using:

- the Exceptional Medical Expenses Act, which covers uninsurable chronic health care services such as home care, day care, and nursing home care

- the Social Support Act, which covers health care services, including day care, that aim to stimulate social participation of vulnerable citizens.

Green care farms have a domestic character, and are mostly small scale. Group size is on average ten people per day. These groups are mostly a mixture of people with dementia and older people who don't have dementia. Green care farms offer free access to outdoor environments (e.g. farmland, garden, orchard, yard) and animals, and a wide range of activities and facilities. In addition to the more conventional day care activities (e.g. leisure and recreational activities), green care farms offer normal domestic and farming activities, such as preparing meals, dish-washing, gardening, feeding animals, sweeping the yard, and going for a walk. Activities can be performed either individually or in groups. Since a wide range of activities is offered at the green care farms, it is likely that people with dementia can find an activity that best fits their preferences and abilities (Figure 6.1). A typical day programme of day care at a green care farm is displayed in Table 6.1.

Most people participating in day care at green care farms have been farmers, have grown up on a farm, live or formerly lived in a rural area, or have affinity with nature and rural life. Green care farms therefore offer opportunities for reminiscence about farming and the outdoors. Green care farms further stimulate the senses of people with dementia through familiar odours (e.g. manure, hay, silage, and food), sounds (e.g. animals, tractors), touch (e.g. animals), and tastes (e.g. raw milk, fresh fruit and vegetables). Green care farms may also help to retain the link with reality through season-related activities and events (e.g. sowing, harvesting, birth of animals) (De Bruin *et al.* 2010b).

Table 6.1 Typical day programme at green care farms

Time	Activity
0930 – 1030	• Arrival of participants at green care farm • Morning tea/coffee • Division of tasks
1030 – 1200	• Participation in preferred activities (e.g. meal preparation, feeding animals, laying the table, getting vegetables from the garden, sweeping the yard, etc.)
1200 – 1300	• Consumption of hot meal
1300 – 1400	• Afternoon nap or participation in activities (e.g. recreational activities or leisure activities: playing games, craft work, going for a walk, reading the newspaper)
1400 – 1430	• Afternoon tea/coffee
1430 – 1600	• Participation in preferred activities: domestic activities (e.g. gardening, making jam out of fruits from orchard); farm activities (e.g. watching and feeding animals); recreational or leisure activities (e.g. sitting outside, playing games, making nest boxes, sanding and painting fences)
1600 – 1630	• Departure of participants

Characteristics of participants of day care at green care farms

People with dementia attending day care at a green care farm are mostly in a relatively early stage of dementia, which is reflected by slight cognitive impairment, slight dependence for activities of daily living, and moderate dependence on instrumental activities of daily living (De Bruin 2009; Schols and Van der Schriek-Van Meel 2006). The average age of people with dementia at green care farms is 78.

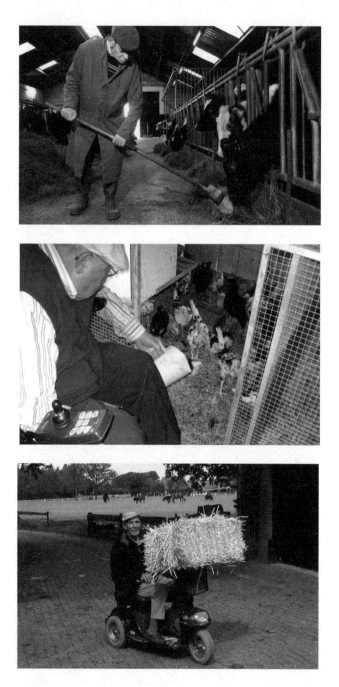

Figure 6.1 Examples of activities of people with dementia attending day care at a green care farm
Photos: Wim and Marga Waanders of green care farm Erve Knippert, Haaksbergen, the Netherlands

It is noteworthy that green care farms seem to serve a different client group from regular day care facilities. Whereas most participants of green care farms are married men with a spouse as their primary caregiver, most participants of day care in regular day care facilities are widowed women with a non-spousal primary caregiver. Additionally, participants in day care at green care farms are on average younger than participants of day care in regular day care facilities (De Bruin 2009).

Quality of care at green care farms

There is as great a heterogeneity among farmers offering green care as there is among the people who use the services of a green care farm. Farmers differ in their motivation for running their farm as a base for health-promoting interventions (e.g. idealism, financial interest, need for challenge, need for personal growth), in their education, and in their personality traits. The extent to which placement of a client is successful will depend on the fit between farmer characteristics, farm characteristics, and client characteristics (including health care demands and personal goals). The different agricultural goals and the various client-related goals require a creative, flexible and individualised approach by the farmers. Personal characteristics of the farmer and the farmer's wife, such as warmth, friendliness, genuineness, openness, empathy, being a good listener, being respectful and being flexible will affect the relationship with the client. The quality of this relationship between the farmer and the client will contribute to the impact of the green care farm environment and the available activities on health outcomes of people with dementia (Enders-Slegers 2008).

It is often thought that farmers and farmers' wives are insufficiently educated to provide health-promoting interventions. For that reason green care farming is sometimes viewed with some scepticism. It appears, however, that farmers' wives in particular often have a professional health care background. Additionally, nowadays some professional schools offer educational programmes to train farmers to become a green care farmer. An increasing number of farmers follow such programmes to learn more about the pathology of their clients and to acquire skills and knowledge to deal accurately with the emotional and behavioural problems of their clients (National Support Centre Agriculture and Care 2011a).

The increasing number of green care farms gave rise to an urgent need for a quality assurance system. To become eligible for the quality mark for green care farms, farmers need to provide insight into their services, activities, protocols, caregivers, complaints service, client records, etc. With this information, potential clients and health care partners can decide whether the health care services provided at the farm match the needs and preferences of clients. Until recently, the quality mark was not compulsory. However, currently there are some discussions going on to make some quality requirements obligatory. In the Netherlands, 75 green care farms are fully awarded the quality mark, and 100 green care farms are in the process of working towards the full award (National Support Centre Agriculture and Care 2011b).

Green care farms versus regular day care facilities

A recent scientific study in the Netherlands compared day programmes where people with dementia participate in day care at green care farms with those of their counterparts participating in day care in regular day care facilities that are mostly affiliated to long-term care institutions (De Bruin 2009). The study showed that both men and women attending day care at a green care farm are more active (i.e. more frequently participating in activities) than their male and female counterparts in regular day care facilities. Activities at green care farms are more diverse than those offered at regular day care facilities. In regular day care facilities activities are mostly limited to recreational and leisure activities such as games and craft work, whereas at green care farms a large variety of normal daily life activities and farm activities are organised in addition (De Bruin et al. 2009). Activities at green care farms are more or less naturally integrated in the environment (e.g. animals need to be fed, crops need to be harvested) and are continuously and simultaneously present, whereas activities in regular day care facilities are not continuously present and need to be introduced one at a time (De Bruin et al. 2010b).

The study additionally showed that people with dementia at green care farms are more frequently outdoors (e.g. garden, forest, yard) or in other buildings belonging to the green care farm (e.g. stable, greenhouse, workshop), whereas people with dementia in regular day care facilities spend almost all day in the same room and indoors. The study further showed that men and women at green care farms are physically more active than their counterparts in regular day care facilities. In regular day care facilities people with dementia are sitting almost all day, whereas at green care farms they are performing activities that require more physical effort for a significantly larger part of the day (De Bruin et al. 2009).

Farming for health

There is a widely-held belief that there is a positive interaction between green care farming and human health. This relationship is, however, difficult to explain and to prove scientifically (Bock and Oosting 2010; De Bruin 2009). Interest in scientific evidence for the potential beneficial health effects of green care farms is growing among farmers, scientists, politicians, health care professionals and potential clients.

A recent Dutch evaluation study showed for which aspects of health of people with dementia green care farms may have beneficial effects (De Bruin 2009; De Bruin *et al.* 2010a). The study showed that participation in day care at green care farms may improve the nutritional status of people with dementia. Older people with dementia attending day care at green care farms had higher energy and fluid intakes than older people with dementia attending regular day care facilities. These findings are of importance, since many older people with dementia are easily prone to malnutrition, weight loss and dehydration (Holm and Soderhamn 2003; White, Pieper, Schmader and Fillenbaum 1996).

The higher activity level of people with dementia at green care farms compared to those attending day care at regular day care facilities may explain the observed differences in dietary intake between people with dementia from both day care settings. Physical activity may lead to an increased energy expenditure and appetite, and therefore to a subsequent higher dietary intake. However, evidence for such an interaction is inconclusive and may explain only part of the observed difference in energy intake. Additional factors may therefore have been responsible for the higher intakes of people with dementia at green care farms, such as the homely eating environment (i.e. the meal is served in dishes, people with dementia can serve themselves, normal cutlery and crockery are used; see Figure 6.2). The social context and environmental ambience are considered to be important factors for dietary intake of older people (De Castro 2002; Gibbons and Henry 2005; Nijs, De Graaf, Kok and Van Staveren 2006). In addition, older people with dementia at green care farms were outdoors more and they were involved in harvesting and preparing meals. Presumably the sight, sound and smell of food being prepared stimulates the appetite in people with dementia, just as they do for most of us (Chalfont 2008).

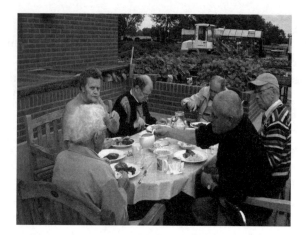

Figure 6.2 Consumption of a hot meal at the green care farm
Photo: Wim and Marga Waanders of green care farm Erve Knippert,
Haaksbergen, the Netherlands

It is expected that green care farms benefit other domains of health,
such as emotional well-being, behaviour and functional performance.
Scientific evidence for these assumptions is, however, not yet available
(De Bruin 2009).

Advantages and disadvantages of green care farms

Green care farming is initiated by farmers and not by the health care
sector. The green care farm environment was seen as rich and challenging
and was therefore considered to be a suitable environment for offering
health-promoting interventions to client groups, including people with
dementia. First, the homely and non-institutional environment at green
care farms may evoke memories and stimulate the senses so that people
with dementia easily feel at home. Second, the variety of environments
at green care farms makes it possible to choose and to participate in
activities that fit the clients' preferences and abilities best. Third, having
a choice may cause a strong sense of autonomy and identity, while the
availability of useful and meaningful activities (e.g. feeding animals,
gardening, preparing meals) may enable people with dementia to feel
useful. Further, the activities offer the opportunity to be together with
other people (e.g. to form bonds, to make new friends) and may offer
distraction and relaxation. Fourth, the opportunities at green care farms
to be active may enhance the mobility of people with dementia.

Green care farms are a successful example of a care service outside the regular health care system, with fewer formalities and regulations. People are more important than rules and regulations. This is an advantage of green care farms, but at the same time a disadvantage, since quality and risk prevention are less controllable. Green care farms operate in a relatively risky environment with regard to accidents and incidents and contagious animal diseases, and some of the farms may not employ professionals in the field of care. One could say that the fact that up to now very few incidents have been reported at green care farms would support the conclusion that this relatively informal care service is very capable of preventing problems because it operates a small-scale and homely setting. However, the trust of the general public only works as long as it lasts.

Green care farms in relation to other current developments in chronic care

The development of green care farms shows a good fit with other current developments in care for people with long-term conditions in the Netherlands. Although the quality of care in Dutch institutions for people with long-term conditions is generally good, some important developments require innovations in the long-term care sector. Over the coming years, the prevalence of chronic illnesses is predicted to increase as a result of the rapid ageing of the world population and the greater longevity of people with long-term conditions. The subsequent increased need for a greater capacity in institutional care, and increasing health care costs, are a concern for health care policymakers. Additionally, there has been a rise in the number of older people who prefer to live at home and adhere to their preferred lifestyles as long as possible, despite their disabilities. These aspects require a challenging reorganisation of the long-term health care sector in the Netherlands, as in many other Western countries facing the same demographic phenomena.

Therefore, in long-term care a gradual ideological shift is taking place. Without minimising the importance of high-quality medical and nursing care, the emphasis is now on improving quality of life by focusing on socialisation or normalisation of long-term care. Socialisation of long-term care aims to enable frail older people (including those with dementia) to live in their own homes or neighbourhoods for as long as possible. This trend requires adapted housing, social services enabling frail older people to participate actively in normal activities as long as possible, and a combination of institutional care services with community care services whenever feasible.

In institutional settings in Western countries, a trend towards socialisation and normalisation is also taking place. For a few years, long-term institutional care has shown a trend of scaling down large institutions to small-scale sheltered housing facilities. These small-scale residences offer people with long-term conditions and frail older people (often people with dementia) a more homely environment. Moreover, these innovative facilities diminish the large institutional atmosphere that so often leads to hospitalisation and loss of autonomy and independence. The same applies for day care services that are offered in Dutch long-term care institutions. Traditionally, the institutional environment of day care facilities affiliated to long-term care institutions is rather artificial. The activities that are provided often do not take the various backgrounds of service users into account and do not correspond well with their normal habits. These disadvantages and the current concept of socialisation for people with long-term conditions have also contributed to changing trends in regular day care facilities. Innovative approaches towards normalisation of regular day care services are taking place and have contributed to the development of day care at green care farms.

Case descriptions
CASE EXAMPLE 1

It is 9.30 am. Taxis have delivered several older people with dementia at the farm. One group participant lives close to the farm and has arrived by bike. After drinking coffee and eating cake – the farmer's wife is celebrating her birthday today – today's tasks are being allocated. Four men, together with a volunteer, will feed the cows, goats, chicken, and rabbits, whereas another man, together with the farmer, will sweep the floor in the stable. The ladies attending day care at the green care farm that day will prepare the hot meal together with the farmer's wife.

CASE EXAMPLE 2

Mrs T was diagnosed with dementia some years ago. She is 75 years old. At home she displays disruptive behaviour, which is extremely demanding and stressful for her husband. Mrs T thinks she is perfectly healthy and was therefore not motivated to attend a service such as regular day care. Moreover, she lives at a farm herself and she thinks that her help is essential there. To convince Mrs T to attend day care at the farm, caregivers at the green care farm have asked her whether she would be willing to do some 'volunteer work' at the farm. This was sufficient to convince Mrs T to come to the green care farm. Currently, she attends day care at the green care farm four times weekly. During these days Mrs T helps with the preparation of the hot meal, cleaning and repairing overalls. She further takes care of the other day care participants by supplying them with coffee. She thinks that she is very busy at the farm, but she is visibly enjoying herself.

CASE EXAMPLE 3

Mr B has been diagnosed with vascular dementia. He feels very uncomfortable about his memory problems and therefore tries to hide these problems. At home he is apathetic; he sits in his chair almost all day. He expresses his incapability with unpleasant behaviour towards his family members. For a few months he has been attending day care at a green care farm three days weekly. At the farm he is very friendly and helpful and whistles as he carries out his duties. At the green care farm there is no continuous need to prove himself and he feels useful. The structure, and the support of the farmer and farmer's wife, help him to perform a large variety of activities. Mr B prefers to help the farmer, by doing tasks like repairing the tools. He mostly goes home in a pleasant mood and his behaviour towards his family members has improved.

CASE EXAMPLE 4

Mr S has Alzheimer's disease. He used to be a carpenter and liked gardening. At home it is very hard to motivate him to participate in any activities. Also, his activities outside the home are gradually lessening. He is, for example, not able to play billiards at his local billiards club anymore. He has been to a regular day care facility in his village once, but he didn't like it there. When Mr S visited a nearby green care farm he was immediately enthusiastic: he became very motivated to work! At the green care farm, he is very active. He participates in a variety of activities: bricklaying, feeding cows and calves, gardening and making nest boxes. Although Mr S's cognitive functioning is declining rapidly, he continues to participate in all the activities.

Acknowledgements

We would like to thank Sylvia Albers of green care farm *De Horst* for providing the case descriptions. All names have been changed to preserve anonymity.

Thanks to Wim and Marga Waanders of green care farm Erve Knippert, Haaksbergen, who provided the photos for this chapter.

References

Bock, B. and Oosting, S. (2010) 'A classification of green care arrangements in Europe.' In J. Dessein and B. Bock (eds) *The Economics of Green Care in Agriculture COST 866.* Loughborough: Loughborough University.

Chalfont, G. (2008) *Design for Nature in Dementia Care.* London: Jessica Kingsley Publishers.

Cohen-Mansfield, J., Lipson, S., Brenneman, K. and Pawlson, L. (2001) 'Health status of participants of adult day care centers.' *Journal of Health and Social Policy 14*, 71–89.

De Bruin, S.R. (2009) 'Sowing in the autumn season: Exploring benefits of green care farms for dementia patients.' PhD thesis, Wageningen University.

De Bruin, S.R., Oosting, S.J., Kuin, Y., Hoefnagels, E.C.M. *et al.* (2009) 'Green care farms promote activity among elderly people with dementia.' *Journal of Housing for the Elderly 23*, 368–389.

De Bruin, S.R., Oosting, S.J., Tobi, H., Blauw, Y.H. *et al.* (2010a) 'Day care at green care farms: A novel way to stimulate dietary intake of community-dwelling older people with dementia?' *Journal of Nutrition, Health and Aging 14*, 5, 352–357.

De Bruin, S.R., Oosting, S.J., Van der Zijpp, A.J., Enders-Slegers, M.J. and Schols, J.M.G.A. (2010b) 'The concept of green care farms for older people with dementia: An integrative framework.' *Dementia 9*, 1, 79–128.

De Castro, J. (2002) 'Age-related changes in the social, psychological, and temporal influences on food intake in free-living, healthy, adult humans.' *Journals of Gerontology: Series A Biological Sciences and Medical Sciences 57*, M368–377.

Droës, R., Meiland, F., Schmitz, M. and Van Tilburg, W. (2004) 'Effect of combined support for people with dementia and carers versus regular day care on behaviour and mood of persons with dementia: Results from a multi-centre implementation study.' *International Journal of Geriatric Psychiatry 19*, 673–684.

Elings, M. and Hassink, J. (2006) 'Farming for Health in the Netherlands.' In J. Hassink and M. Van Dijk (eds) *Farming for Health.* Wageningen: Springer.

Enders-Slegers, M. J. (2008) 'Therapeutic farming or therapy on a farm?' In J. Dessein (ed.) *Farming for Health. Proceedings of the Community of Practice Farming for Health.* Ghent: ILVO.

Gibbons, M. and Henry, C. (2005) 'Does eating environment have an effect on food intake in the elderly?' *The Journal of Nutrition, Health and Aging 9*, 25–29.

Hassink, J. and Van Dijk, M. (2006) 'Farming for health across Europe: Comparison between countries, and recommendations for a research policy agenda.' In J. Hassink and M. Van Dijk (eds) *Farming for Health.* Wageningen: Springer.

Hassink, J., Zwartbol, C., Agricola, H.J., Elings, M. and Thissen, J.T.N.M. (2007) 'Current status and potential of care farms in the Netherlands.' *NJAS Wageningen Journal of Life Sciences 55*, 21–36.

Haubenhofer, D., Elings, M., Hassink, J. and Hine, R. (2010) 'The development of green care in Western European countries.' *Explore 6*, 106–111.

Hine, R. (2008) 'Care farming in the UK: Recent findings and implications.' In J. Dessein (ed.) *Farming for Health. Proceedings of the Community of Practice Farming for Health.* Ghent: ILVO.

Hine, R., Peacock, J. and Pretty, J. (2008) 'Care farming in the UK: contexts, benefits and links with therapeutic communities.' *Therapeutic Communities 29*, 245–260.

Holm, B. and Soderhamn, O. (2003) 'Factors associated with nutritional status in a group of people in an early stage of dementia.' *Clinical Nutrition I*, 385–389.

Jarrott, S.E, Zarit, S.H., Berg, S. and Johansson, L. (1998) 'Adult day care for dementia: A comparison of programs in Sweden and the United States.' *Journal of Cross-Cultural Gerontology 13*, 99–108.

National Support Centre Agriculture and Care (2011a) 'Erkende opleiding voor zorgboeren.' Accessed on 27 October 2010 at www.landbouwzorg.nl/nieuwsbrieven/nieuwsbrief_5.html.

National Support Centre Agriculture and Care (2011b) *Kwaliteitswaarborg Zorgboerderijen.* [Online] Accessed on 10 January 2011 at www.landbouwzorg.nl/index.php?pagid=38.

Nijs, K., De Graaf, C., Kok, F. and Van Staveren, W. (2006) 'Effect of family style mealtimes on quality of life, physical performance and body weight of nursing home residents: Cluster randomised controlled trial.' *British Medical Journal 332*, 1180–1184.

Roest, A., Oltmer, K., Driest, P. and Jans, A. (2010) 'Thuis op de zorgboerderij. Handreiking kleinschalig wonen voor ouderen met dementie.' Taskforce Multifunctionele Landbouw. LEI-Wageningen UR: Vilans.

Schols, J.M.G.A. and Van Der Schriek-Van Meel, C. (2006) 'Day care for demented elderly in a diary farm setting: Positive first impressions.' *Journal of the American Medical Directors Association 7*, 456–459.

White, H., Pieper, C., Schmader, K. and Fillenbaum, G. (1996) 'Weight change in Alzheimer's disease.' *Journal of the American Geriatrics Society 44*, 265–72.

Working Group on the Health Benfits of Green Care, COST 866 (2010) 'Green Care: A Conceptual Framework.' In J. Sempik, R. Hine and D.W. Hine (eds) *Green Care: A Conceptual Framework.* Loughborough: Loughborough University.

Chapter 7

No Roof but the Sky Above My Head

JAMES MCKILLOP

I led an ordinary life and was forever out on my pushbike, travelling all over the country. When I was 18, I cycled from Wishaw in Lanarkshire down to London and back. I was out on the bike every day. When at home, I spent hours in the garden. I stayed with my mother, and I cultivated plants you could eat, with some space for flowers. I liked to gather cuttings from other gardeners. The soil was fertile and I could grow just about anything. Living near a farm, good manure was available. I did not go to pubs or discos. I preferred being out in the open. I could enjoy just sitting on the doorstep in the evening, watching the plants grow. I could also talk to passers-by. I also walked for miles, and was lucky to stay near the country. The sky and I were constant companions. But I got older and took ill.

In the year before I was diagnosed with dementia, I stayed in my house. It wasn't a home any more, as family life was unbearable. My wife and children didn't speak to me anymore. This was because I had behavioural problems, and didn't appreciate I had them. I had changed into a tyrant. (Getting back outside into the community and with the help of medication, that, thankfully, is no longer the case.)

I sat alone in the living room, staring at a blank TV screen. I couldn't even be bothered to switch it on. I didn't read or do anything, I just sat and stared and brooded. I was deeply depressed. It got to the stage where I didn't bathe myself, shave or change clothes, without being pressured by my wife. If she got my clothes off me, when she went to work, I would go to the washing basket and put my old clothes back on. My daughter called me an old Jakey (Scottish word for a dirty, unkempt down-and-out).

A diagnosis changed quite a few things. My wife, now knowing I had an illness, became more understanding and a comfort to me. My children came round and started to speak to me. They listened to my advice and did the opposite. How wise they were!

But I was still in the doldrums. I had met people in the advanced stages of dementia many times, when I worked in large mental health hospitals, and I saw myself being like that any day now. My life was turned upside down.

I couldn't get it out of my head that I was doomed. Then I met someone – Brenda, from Alzheimer Scotland. She came to do a one-off interview, for me to claim benefits. It wasn't her job to do anything else but send in the form and go to the next client. However, she must have seen a want in me. She invited me to help at a stall selling items to raise funds for dementia. I didn't want to leave the safety of the house, but she has a way with her, not taking no for an answer. When I gave in and said I would come, but I could not handle money, she replied I could do what I could manage. A little goes a long way.

I was a bit nervous about going outside, the open air seemed threatening. Anyway, I made a great effort, girded my loins, scrubbed up and off I went. I was surprised, when standing at the stall, that I could speak again, and respond to people. Months of non-communication orally, had left its mark on me. Yet here I was speaking. I marvelled at myself.

Brenda didn't let up. She got me a support worker, Marilyn, who would take me out in her car, several hours a week. By coincidence, or was it part of Brenda's scheming, Marilyn was a great photographer. She retrained me in how to use my manual camera, a Nikkormat FT3, and we took photographs wherever we went (see Figure 7.1 on page 89). I enjoyed being out in the fresh air and the delightful company. My brain started ticking over again. It seemed to work in conjunction with the drugs I was taking. I slowly began to look forward to my trips to that world outside what was now a home again, a place to return to for a welcome from the family and cats.

Through time, I began to venture out by myself. This brought its own problems. I still thought as a driver, and when a filter light came on at junctions, I would stride out and was nearly knocked over several times. I had even more toots from angry drivers. I used to shake my fist at them as I thought they were in the wrong. It took time to adjust to becoming a pedestrian. I also had trouble with buses. I couldn't count out the exact change and I got Maureen, my beloved wife, to count money into wee plastic bags for me. However, I still had problems. I would take only enough for the journey there, and forget I had a return journey, and had to walk home on many an occasion. Well, it did my figure good. Thank goodness I now have a bus pass.

I became addicted to going out and became uneasy and unsettled when confined to my home, yes it was still a home, such as when the weather was icy. I began to appreciate that to enjoy my sense of well-being, I needed a good balance between being out in the community and staying at home to follow my hobbies, such as reading. I now find contentment reading every day, after a trip to the other world.

I have not mentioned confidence yet. Many people, and through no fault of their own, lose confidence after diagnosis. Mine had been shattered, but it was built back up again. To cut a long story short, I have regained the confidence to enjoy the outdoors. Communicating with mother nature, on a one-to-one basis. We had lost touch for so long. It was great to be back.

It can be daunting for some people to venture outdoors, even into the garden. But with good company, it can be rewarding, seeing the seasons unfold. The snowdrops and crocuses in spring, followed by tulips and daffodils and other flowers as the year progresses. I feel they put on their finery for us to enjoy, and I appreciate and enjoy the display. They never fail to appear each year, even after a hard winter. Poets sing their praises, and who can forget the Wordsworth image of daffodils fluttering and dancing in the breeze? Robert Burns compared his love to a rose.

Actors sing to the trees in the musical *Paint Your Wagon*. And who has not sent or received a red rose on Valentine's day?

It can be peaceful and cathartic, just sitting in a garden in the sunshine, with a good book and a glass of what you fancy by your side. Chocolates, cakes and biscuits also go down well. And it doesn't have to be daylight. If you wrap up well, or have a garden heater, you can stay warm for so long. If you choose some plants, such as night-stock, they release their fragrant perfume as night falls, and the sensation can help you relax before sleep. The stars come out to mesmerise me with their winking, and keep me company. The moon does his bit too, and I don't know who watches who. He puts on funny shapes for me, to keep track of the days. In colder weather he puts on a full display to warn me of possible frost.

I was on respite in the country, and it was sunny but frosty. I put on my warmest fleece, grasped a cup of warm coffee and savoured the atmosphere. I could listen to small birds singing their souls out for me, something I can't do at home in a city.

If you have young children or grandchildren, a garden can provide endless hours of fun. Weeds, detested by adults, can entertain the young ones. Making daisy chains, blowing seeded dandelions to tell the time, or making perfume from petals, especially the rose petal variety.

Snow blankets the ground in winter, but it can be fun for children to leave their footprints in the snow and build snowmen. But you can look forward to the spring, when blossom decks the trees and carpets the ground white or pink, as it falls. Children like to scatter the corolla. When autumn arrives, it is great to see them running, scattering the fallen leaves, and hearing them rustle. Alas, it is work for us adults, but we were young once.

I have little experience of courtyards, but I can recommend one. It is at the back of the Garrison in Millport on the Isle of Cumbrae (reached by ferry, no senior discounts) or by bus (concession cards accepted) from Largs. You need a good day of course, but when sunny, it is a suntrap. Remember your suncream/sunglasses. The cafeteria is yards away and your dog can come with you and have a drink from a bowl of water in the courtyard. Small birds come, seeking crumbs from your plate, and brazenly hop up to your feet.

A domino effect happened to others who labour in the community. Walking again meant work for the cobbler. Café owners such as at One Seven Ate welcomed me as a regular customer. The chemist sold me cream to protect me from the sun's rays. The bicycle shop in Millport hired me a bike (and one for Maureen). Jessops sold me new cameras and memory cards and gave back-up advice when my memory failed me. My favourite charity shops provided me with a supply of books and CDs. I couldn't do all this imprisoned in four walls.

The outdoors is for living in, working in and socialising in, and paves the way for a pleasant evening by the fireside. There is no charge (as yet) to step outside, breathe in and savour life's rich tapestries.

Epilogue

James continues to go outdoors and enjoy life. However, due to osteoarthritis he cannot walk as far and for as long as he used to. But on the bright side, this allows him more quality time in places he visits and more time for an extra cuppa. And more time to absorb his surroundings. He likes going to Whitelee wind-farm (near Eaglesham) to sit indoors/ outdoors depending on the weather, mesmerised by the windmill blades lazily turning, sipping a cappuccino and reflecting on good times. The fresh air blows the cobwebs away.

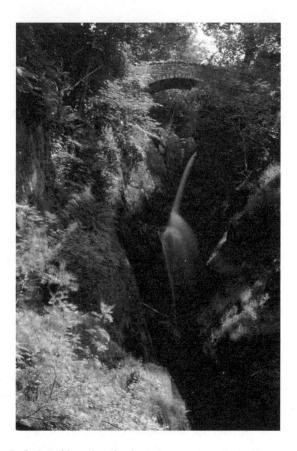

Figure 7.1 The fresh air blows the cobwebs away
Photo: James McKillop

Chapter 8

Animal-Assisted Activities for People Living with Dementia

MARCUS FELLOWS AND ANN RAINSFORD

The concept of animals, and pets in particular, within the home having a positive effect on people with either mental or physical illness is not a new idea. We can look back to the work of Florence Nightingale in the mid-nineteenth century who advocated using animals in nursing and noted the benefit of a small animal for chronically sick people. There have been therapeutic communities involving animals since the ninth century in Belgium, and since 1792 in the UK. The UK Retreat used rabbits and birds to encourage psychiatric patients to care for animals. A centre for the treatment of epilepsy was founded in Germany in 1867 and by 1984 had 5000 residents utilising animal-assisted activities (AAA) through birds, cats, dogs, horses, farm animals and a wild game park (Dawson and Campbell 2005).

In psychotherapy Boris Levinson (1969) first documented case studies in which his dog Jingles worked as a co-therapist in his US clinic. Levinson's work, originally termed 'pet-facilitated therapy' (since replaced by AAA/AAT to indicate reciprocal relationships rather than a passive pet) is generally thought to have signalled the origins of animals in contemporary therapy.

AAA and people with dementia

Some documented or research programmes of AAA/AAT have involved people with dementia. Studies have found that the presence of a dog for people with dementia increases social interactions, smiles and laughter (e.g. see Batson *et al.* 1998; Verderber 1991). Beyersdorfer and Birkenhauer (1990) reported people with dementia to be calmer when therapy dogs visited. Edwards and Beck (2002) found that people with dementia ate more and gained weight when eating in a room with an aquarium, in a study over a 16-week period. Baun and McCabe (2003) examined the therapeutic benefit for people with dementia of adopting a dog, and speculated about the potential to train dogs to alert carers to dangers for the person. Tribet, Boucharlet and Myslinski (2008) found many psychological benefits in a French dog therapy programme involving three people with dementia over a nine-month period. These included calming, increased self-esteem, increased interaction with dogs, and saying that the dog was affectionate and that they could identify themselves with the dog.

The difficulty of comparing studies in the AAA and AAT range of programmes is the small scale of many of the studies, and inconsistencies both in design of the programmes and in the way they are recorded and reported. This was also highlighted by Perkins (2008) who reviewed studies using dog-assisted therapy with groups of people with dementia (ranging from four to 28). They found a number of difficulties with comparing the studies and were critical of the way they had been conducted and recorded. They also suggested that the positive outcomes reported for AAT might equally have been achieved by the introduction of any novel activity, and could certainly be affected by the presence of a human dog-handler.

Filan and Llewellyn-Jones (2006) reviewed studies of AAT for people with dementia to consider the impact on their behavioural and psychological symptoms. They found that several studies suggested a reduction in aggression and agitation and an increase in social behaviour of people with dementia when a dog is present. They did not limit their review to dogs but also included a study of robotic pets, cats and the aquarium study already mentioned. They raise the issue of resident reaction to visiting animals and the positive effect of pet interaction on staff and carers. They also point to the lack of conclusions on the duration of the beneficial effects of AAT.

Neville Williams House: A case study

Background

Neville Williams House is a registered nursing care home owned and managed by BCOP (Broadening Choices for Older People). The home has a total of 50 residents, the majority of whom have varying degrees of dementia; some of the people with more serious impairments are accommodated in a specialist care environment where staff time devoted to the residents is more intensive than in the remaining parts of the home.

The home also offers a day care facility for people with dementia as part of a support service for both individuals and their carers.

BCOP had been involved in AAA/AAT for some years in all of its care homes, relying on visiting charities and individuals who brought dogs or cats to the home for what had become termed 'petting' therapy for many of the residents. The basis of the introduction of animals was very much centred on community integration, bringing the 'outside' world into the home, where institutional isolation may become a problem. It was also recognised by some staff that both dogs and cats have a calming effect on some residents, while with others they stimulate discussions about their own pets and the experiences they had with them earlier in their lives.

The decision to take the concept of animal activity, and what benefits may be brought about by widening the scope of the activities, was made following a chance discussion and visit to the Netherlands, where AAA is supported by both local government and the medical profession.

Early days

In January 2009 BCOP identified Neville Williams House as a suitable home to establish what has become known as the 'animal farm'. The decision was based on a number of factors which were to influence the planned outcomes, but in essence required the following:

1. Appropriate space to house the animals.

2. Staff who would commit to the project.

3. Support from the trustees, both financial and conceptual.

1. APPROPRIATE SPACE TO HOUSE THE ANIMALS

The plan was to introduce animals that would in the main live outside in the grounds of the home, but at the same time could come into the building and be a part of the environment and care.

Neville Williams House is a long building that runs parallel to the road, with a long and relatively narrow back garden above a short, steep slope to the fence below. The steep slope was unusable by the residents until a long sloping path was carved out of it from right to left. This made space for animal accommodation on both sides, fenced off from the path to allow optimal viewing. Near the foot of the path a water feature was installed, so water runs down the slope in a set of small falls and there is a pond at the foot with fish in it. Another larger pond is under construction at the top of the slope. There is a free-standing large aviary near the conservatory in the garden and two fish tanks inside the home.

Small animals (e.g. rabbits and guinea pigs) were amongst the first to be housed, followed by chickens and ducks. Within two months aviary birds were introduced along with Kune Kune pigs and pygmy goats (Figure 8.1). There are also a lot of bird tables, bird feeders and bird boxes within sight of the conservatory and lounges.

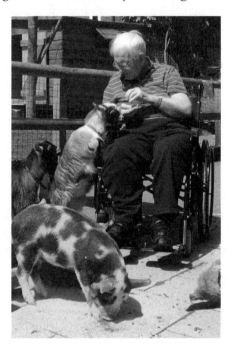

Figure 8.1 A resident feeds some of the animals at Neville Williams House
Photo: Peter Jones, Community image

The choice and selection of the animals was made with care. The farm did not happen without careful attention to factors such as potential risk. This has been minimised with careful fencing, careful choice of animals (the goats, for example, are a breed known for their mild temperament and they are castrated to ensure that they remain so). Support and advice are provided by the local vet, the dealers and the Birmingham Nature Centre. Local animal experts and government departments also proved invaluable when dealing with the mountains of 'red tape' associated with the project.

Interestingly most residents turned out to have had some experience of animals even though this home is in a very urban area. Many of them had parents with small-holdings, others went to farms for their holidays or had been evacuated to farms during World War II. Many had had chickens during the war. Many had pets. Others had had periods of their lives when they lived in the country. Cats are not part of the farm since they are the one animal to which one resident had an aversion. (No other resident had any problems with any of the animals, birds or fish.)

2. STAFF
The nursing home was fortunate to have a gardener with both a passion for and experience of rearing animals and birds. Her family had reared poultry and she herself had dogs and birds. She had to learn about pigs and goats. She was responsible for the care of all the animals and birds. She had a back-up member of staff who took over when she was off duty or on leave. She was also the main staff member responsible for linking the animals and birds with the residents. She took the rabbits into the most impaired residents' lounge, for example, and placed them on the knees of the seated residents, where they sat comfortably, being stroked. She also took residents to the pigs, who loved being scratched. Many residents like to scatter corn for the chickens and to collect the eggs. Another staff member has now taken over these responsibilities. The next birds to be introduced will be a couple of parrots, which will live in a large cage in the entrance hall. A lot of the AAA are weather-dependent, with a great deal more activity in the summer months. Bird tables and feeders are, of course, visible and active all year round. A basement corridor is currently being decorated by the residents with a relief of the animals and birds so that there is something to look at, and touch, when the weather is inclement.

3. SUPPORT FROM THE TRUSTEES
The trustees needed to invest in the initial construction project of the path, fences and animal and bird accommodation, as well as in the animals and birds themselves. Investment continues in the parrot cage and second fish pond. The project has been so successful that it is being rolled out to other BCOP nursing homes. The ongoing costs are not great, since the animals which are chosen are hardy and, in the main, live outside.

Benefits

Like most of the research and studies carried out in respect of animal activities and the benefits to people living with dementia, the home has had some difficulty in measuring benefit in a structured and evidence-based way. It has become clear to staff, residents and relatives that anecdotal evidence can be produced showing that residents' level of activity and general well-being has improved – in some cases by as much as 50 per cent if measured against initial care planning documentation, while others have seen minor improvement. However, due to the relatively short period the project has been in existence, coupled with the lack of useful measurable information provided to the staff when residents first enter the home, and the short duration some residents' stay, it can be argued that the accuracy of the benefit outcomes is questionable. It can also be argued that the improvements seen in some residents could be attributed to other factors in the home (e.g. the introduction of a structured care package which was lacking prior to their change of environment). Recognising such shortcomings, it is nevertheless felt by all of those involved in the project that the following can be identified as benefits to some degree, to both residents and the staff and management of the home.

MENTAL STIMULATION

As part of the normal assessment procedure when new residents enter the home, staff work with both the resident and their advocates to gain an understanding of their cognitive skills, to enable them to develop a package of care tailored to the individual needs of the resident. The assessment is recorded and reviewed on a regular basis, noting changes as and when they occur.

Staff have noted that those residents who take an active part in the AAA show a greater degree of awareness and improved communication skills during the activity – more so than when they are involved in other activities such as art and craft work. It has further been noted that for some residents, both staff and family members have observed improvement in cognitive skills over a period of time, and this is also confirmed by the regular care assessments carried out within the home. It is, however, accepted that this improvement may be the result of more than just the influence of the animal activity, and only further detailed research will be able to confirm what elements of the change may be due to AAA.

PHYSICAL CHANGES

Physical capabilities are also assessed when residents enter the home, with a view to creating a package of care that works to improve the physical well-being of the resident. While the assessment is not scientific, it follows standard practice. Again, this is done in conjunction with the resident and advocates. As with cognitive changes, any physical change is recorded as part of the regular planning for the individual.

As AAA does require residents to use the grounds of the home, the majority of physical interaction and engagement with animals is carried out on a one-to-one basis which requires greater movement on the part of the resident (e.g. feeding and 'petting' the animals). Collecting hens' eggs involves both physical activity and ownership of the animals and associated activity.

Staff have also noticed the efforts made by residents who are less physically able, to adapt the scope of their own abilities in the way they interact with the animals. Stroking the pigs, for example, is done with feet and toes, rather than the conventional hand stroking, by residents who are wheelchair-reliant. Because of the increased use of their limbs, residents have become more agile and flexible, achieving the optimum movement they have available to them. This in turn has helped some of the residents deal with the mental issues associated with loss of movement.

As with the cognitive improvements, it is fair to say the same caveats apply, in that data cannot substantiate evidence to suggest that all of the improvements are due to AAA. (The home provides a number of physical therapies which aid improvement for all residents.) However, residents who take a more physical part in the animal activity do appear to show greater improvements in a shorter period.

REDUCTION OF SOCIAL ISOLATION

One of the unforeseen and measurable benefits of the animal project has been the reduction of isolation problems experienced by many residents in institutional care. It is fair to say that the majority of homes make every effort to provide activities that take residents out of the home and into the 'community'. It is also fair to say that a good deal of feedback from residents and advocates suggests that more 'outings' are requested but rarely provided, due primarily to the financial cost of providing additional carers and transport.

While the animal project does not in any way replace the need for community activity, it has brought many more people into an environment that was previously seen by some (particularly younger children) as 'not a very nice place to visit'. The animal project has increased visitor numbers by over 50 per cent in the past 12 months alone, with a noticeable increase in younger members of the community and families. As one resident commented, 'I see more of my great-grandchildren now than I ever did before I moved into here.'

Benefit conclusions

The project is still very much in its infancy and the benefits are in the main seen anecdotally, in that it has been difficult to prove beyond doubt that AAA is responsible for the benefits outlined above. It is clear that more research is needed to enable further development of the AAA project, but for as long as residents and advocates confirm that the quality of life improves for themselves and others, the home will continue to provide and develop the activity.

A way forward

While it is recognised that a number of research projects have been undertaken looking at how interaction with animals has helped people with cognitive and physical impairment, very little research has concentrated on institutional settings and improvements made in such environments. BCOP has continued to argue that the benefits can far outweigh the cost in staff time and financial input. However, if they are to achieve their objective, by enabling a wider audience to benefit from AAA, BCOP recognises the need to provide more objective evidence. To this end, with the help of the Dementia Services Development Centre at Stirling University, a grant has been secured to carry out a three-year research project looking specifically at AAA for people with dementia. It is hoped that, following on from this research, a 'toolkit' can be developed that will enable other providers to establish their own activity programme with the backing of 'best practice' models.

Acknowledgements

The animal-assisted therapy at Neville Williams House would not have been possible without the dedicated help of many staff in the home, some of whom also assisted with information for this chapter.

References

Batson, K., McCabe, B., Baun, M.M. and Wilson, C. (1998) 'The effect of a therapy dog on socialization and physiological indicators of stress in persons diagnosed with Alzheimer's Disease.' In C.C. Wilson and D.C. Turner (eds) *Companion Animals in Human Health.* London: Sage.

Baun, M.M. and McCabe, B.W. (2000) 'The Role Animals Play in Enhancing Quality of Life for the Elderly.' In A. Fine (ed.) *Handbook on Animal-Assisted Therapy: Theoretical Foundations and Guidelines for Practice.* London: Academic Press.

Baun, M.M. and McCabe, B.W. (2003) 'Companion animals and persons with dementia of the Alzheimer's type: Therapeutic possibilities.' *American Behavioral Scientist 47,* 1, 42–51.

Beyersdorfer, P.S. and Birkenhauer, D.M. (1990) 'The therapeutic use of pets on an Alzheimer's unit.' *American Journal of Alzheimer's Disease and Other Dementias 5,* 1, 13–17.

Dawson, S. and Campbell, B. (2005) 'Animal-Assisted Therapy and Animal-Assisted Activities.' In J.-A. Dono and E. Ormerod (eds) *Older People and Pets.* Burford: Society for Companion Animal Studies.

Edwards, N.E. and Beck, A. (2002) 'Animal-assisted therapy and nutrition in Alzheimer's disease.' *Western Journal of Nursing Research 24,* 6, 697–712.

Filan, S.L. and Llewellyn-Jones, R.H. (2006) 'Animal-assisted therapy for dementia: a review of the literature.' *International Psychogeriatrics 18,* 4, 597–611.

Levinson, B. (1969) *Pet-oriented Child Psychotherapy.* Springfield, IL: Charles C. Thomas.

Perkins, J. (2008) 'Dog assisted therapy for older people with dementia: A review.' *Australasian Journal on Ageing 27,* 4, 177–182.

Tribet, J., Boucharlat, M. and Myslinski, M. (2008) 'Animal-assisted therapy for people suffering from severe dementia.' *Encephale 34,* 2, 183–186.

Verderber, S. (1991) Elderly person's appraisal of animals in the residential environment.' *Anthrozoos 4,* 164–173.

Chapter 9

Gardening and Dementia

MEMBERS OF THE PARK CLUB AND RACHAEL LITHERLAND

> If I couldn't go outside into the garden, I'd die. I like fresh air
> on my face. I like to battle the breeze. I watch the birds. I see
> the seasons.
>
> *Person with dementia*

Gardens have been perceived as a source of pleasure and a place for
meditation and relaxation for many centuries. A garden serves to promote
the activity and health of body, mind and spirit (Sempik, Aldridge and
Becker 2003).

For people with dementia, access to and enjoyment of gardens can
become limited. Larner (2005) suggests that a range of cognitive abilities
are necessary for successful gardening:

- *Memory*: for shapes, colours, and names of plants.

- *Visuo-spatial skills*: for the layout of borders and arranging plants,
  flowers and vegetables.

- *Praxis*: for the handling of plants and garden implements.

- *Executive function*: interest in the subject and ability to plan ahead.

The impact of dementia on these cognitive abilities may result in a long-
standing gardener losing interest in gardening or not having the abilities
to garden in the way that he or she once had. This personal experience
can be compounded by physical difficulties in accessing a garden, caused
by disability or by moving to a care setting where spending time in a
garden is not encouraged or supported.

The enjoyment of gardens and the activity of gardening has been
promoted as being of real benefit to people with dementia. Chaplin
(2003) discusses gardening as a form of occupational therapy for people
with dementia; gardens provide a source of multi-sensory stimulation and
therapeutic value – 'feeling better' when involved with a garden (Sempik,
Aldridge and Becker 2003). Gardening has also been shown to impact on

health and well-being; for example, Lee and Kim (2007) concluded that indoor gardening was found to be effective for improved sleep, decreased agitation and enhanced cognition of people with dementia.

Enhancing the healing environment

A National Health Service team in Devon is the recipient of a national grant programme to improve a hospital environment for people with dementia. The programme supports local health care professionals to work in partnership with service users to improve the environment in which they deliver care.

The design of an accessible and dementia-appropriate garden is central to the rebuild programme. What better way to design a dementia-appropriate space than to engage people with dementia in the process?

Three small group discussions were organised at a specialist day centre for people with dementia in Exeter, Devon, with nine people involved in total. Additionally, three people shared their experiences and ideas in one-to-one discussions.

Most participants were able to engage in some way with the discussion topic. One man who was very embarrassed about his word-finding problems and apologised frequently in the early parts of his discussion became very animated as he remembered his gardening experiences, and subsequently began to talk more fluently and with less embarrassment. One discussion with two women took place with views over a local park where the women had just been for a walk. Visual props were used to help other people to engage in conversation. These included:

- a selection of pictures from *In the Garden – In Pictures* (a 'Pictures to Share' publication)
- sprigs of rosemary and lavender
- a quince
- a pulled beetroot complete with roots and soil
- a watering can
- packets of seeds.

The remainder of this chapter is handed over to people with dementia. Their voices describe personal gardening experiences as they reflect on the benefits and impact of gardens and gardening on their lives.

Experiencing the elements

Gardening, for many, was about having opportunity to be out of doors, and to experience the weather and its impact on the garden and oneself.

'I like to get out into the garden – feeling the fresh air. You need to breathe it.'

'I'd rather be out than in.'

'I love to go into my garden when it is wet outside, raining. To feel the rain on my face – there is nothing like it.'

'Mud, I love it. When your feet touch the ground and they go "squelch"…'

'I like to see trees. I quite like walking through a forest. I like a big scale.'

'I like to put my fingers right through the grass. Always goes through my nose. You can smell the outdoor life.'

Importantly, wet weather conditions were described more than warm weather, with people vividly describing the sensations of wind, rain and mud.

Working the land

Seven of the people with dementia had been avid gardeners in their time. They remembered the physical aspects of gardening, the connection with the land and the joy of growing.

'Oh, feeling the soil between my fingers. Dirt under my nails – that smell. You know you are alive.'

'A greenhouse – you need a greenhouse. Tomatoes – I like to eat them from a greenhouse. They are a different flavour, the ones you've grown yourself. They smell different.'

'Herbs – things you can smell – that's what I like to grow.'

'I like to grow things that are natural – bluebells, flowers that are in season, honeysuckle and daisies.'

'You forget everything when you are out there. It's just you and your spade.'

Of the seven, no one was still an active gardener. Some people had moved and no longer had a garden. Others now paid 'professionals' to tend their gardens, sharing in small decisions such as the choice of plants.

Appreciating the gardening cycle

A few people touched upon changes in season and the differences in gardens at different times of the year. The continual cycle of growth and decline and growth was referred to, and so was the relevance that this has for day-to-day life.

> 'I love flowers – flowers at different times of the year. You have to know what you are doing, to plant them in at the right time. You have to put the right plants in for each season.'

> 'I like to watch the garden grow. To see things grow and then start again. I like to see it coming up.'

> 'You see life out there. Everything has its time.'

Reaping the rewards of hard work

The sheer graft of gardening was mentioned by a lot of people, but so were the positive feelings this instils. People expressed memories of the improved taste of produce from their gardens, usually as a consequence of the efforts they put into their garden.

> 'My garden is what I have made it. It is a social place – everyone comes from all around to look at my garden. It's the first thing they used to do – let's have a look and see what you've been up to. I used to do it all, vegetables, the lot. I'd feed the house. I leave it to the real experts now. But I still go to the garden centres to choose the flowers – they make a lovely job. I tell them what I want. It is lovely sitting out the back with seats you can fold.'

> 'I like putting plants in and chucking them out. It's all part of tidying up.'

> 'I had it all – pear trees, apple trees. There is nothing like growing and picking your own. You know you did it.'

> 'I get the fidgets if I sit too long.'

> 'I like a bit of a potter. I couldn't do it all now [gardening].'

'When you come in at the end of the day all tired, you know you have done a good job.'

No one was still actively gardening but these comments, mostly made in the present tense and with great animation, suggest a real connection with the activity of gardening and the remembered personal benefits.

'Being'

For many people the garden had become a source of pleasure and relaxation. The garden provided an opportunity to just 'be' and appreciate, activating all the senses.

'I like to see it [the garden] coming up.'

'I don't do it any more [grow vegetables]. I like to sit in it now.'

'I like to smell the garden.'

'The garden has to be peaceful. It's no good having a cat around!'

'Water – ripple, ripple. It should be moving, not staying still.'

'Hearing birds singing. But it shouldn't be too quiet. Birds don't like it too quiet.'

Loss of a garden

Some people were able to reflect on the changes that age and dementia had brought in their relationship with their gardens.

'I used to grow vegetables – enough for the house. Not any more. I wouldn't know where to start.'

'I like to see it coming up – but I don't touch it now.'

'Helping out in a garden is good. But I wouldn't want to ruin it.'

'I've really enjoyed talking about this. I'd forgotten how much I loved my garden.'

Conclusions

In their discussions this small group of people with dementia reconnected with their personal experiences of gardens and gardening. Although people were not invited to take part in the discussion because of any expressed interest in gardening, nine out of ten participants did in fact have a very real interest (one woman preferred bracing sea walks!) either in appreciating a garden or actively contributing to a garden.

Some people recalled, with enthusiasm, their own gardening experiences and the impact this had on their lives. Unfortunately no one was still actively gardening, although many people had opportunity to appreciate a garden and outdoor space.

If we refer back to Larner's (2005) list at the beginning of this chapter, it would seem that the cognitive changes that people's dementia brings (plus the ageing process more generally) can impact substantially on ability, willingness and access to ongoing gardening activity. However, the strong recollections of feelings, smells and sights associated with people's individual experiences suggests that they retain an emotional connection to gardens and gardening that, with the right support, could be nurtured and could grow again.

References

Chaplin, R. (2003) 'Occupational therapy interventions.' In R. Baldwin and M. Murray (eds) *Younger People with Dementia. A Multidisciplinary Approach.* London: Martin Dunitz.

Larner, A.J. (2005) 'Gardening and dementia.' *International Journal of Geriatric Psychiatry* 20, 8, 796–797.

Lee, Y. and Kim, S. (2007) 'Effects of indoor gardening on sleep, agitation and cognition in dementia patients – a pilot study.' *International Journal of Geriatric Psychiatry 23*, 5, 485–489.

Pictures to Share (2008) *In the Garden – In Pictures.* Peckforton: Pictures to Share.

Sempik, J., Aldridge, J. and Becker, S. (2003) '*Social and therapeutic horticulture: Evidence and messages from research.*' (Literature review.) Loughborough: CCFR.

Chapter 10

Allotments

LORRAINE ROBERTSON

Alzheimer Scotland delivers day care services and home support services across West Dunbartonshire. The service has a day care facility based in the centre of Dumbarton. The area covered by the service consists of three towns, Alexandria, Dumbarton and Clydebank, as well as several villages in more rural settings.

The service supports between 65 and 85 people with dementia, their carers and families, on a weekly basis. The average age is 82 years old, although a tiny minority are under 65. There are 60 day care places, 300 hours home support, two drop-in sessions and two community arts-based activity sessions every week.

The service has a large allotment, near to the day centre, which is rented from the local authority and is a short, five minute walk from the centre building.

When the opportunity arose to rent the allotment, it was discussed at a meeting with the people who are supported by the service. Several of those with dementia said that they had previous experience of working on their own allotments, or that they had lived on farms when children. Some who had experienced the war years remembered having vegetable plots and helping to produce their own food. It was agreed that having an allotment would be of great benefit and would be widely enjoyed.

When we first had access to the allotment space it was wild and overgrown. We would have to start from scratch. We were fortunate in having a couple of volunteers who were able to undertake the heavy work of clearing the ground. The next stage was to plan the layout of the allotment to maximise the use of the space and ground and to ensure as much access as possible.

The access to the allotment is along a grassy path which runs along the bottom of all the allotment plots on the site. It is possible to access the allotment with a wheelchair when the ground is hard; however, this is not possible when the ground is soft. As the area is the property of the local authority it has not been possible to improve the access without the cooperation of the council. We are looking at the possibility of alternative access from the rear of the service allotment, which backs onto a hardcore path.

The allotment (see Figure 10.1) has a large garden shed for the storage of equipment and for activities like re-potting. There is also a large greenhouse and this is used for propagating seedlings, growing tomatoes and peppers and strawberries, and sitting down to have a cup of tea when it is raining.

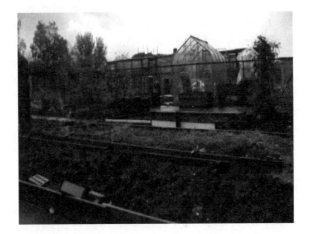

Figure 10.1 The allotment: A general view
Photo: Lorraine Robertson

A part of the space was sectioned off and paved to create an outdoor seating area. A garden table and chairs were purchased through a specific donation. This allows those with physical impariments to participate, and it also offers the opportunity for comfortable rest periods.

There are ground-level beds in which we grow potatoes, cabbages, carrots and turnips. Raised beds are used for growing peas and onions. A herb garden was also created at a higher access level. Some of the border areas are used to grow different types of flowers. Several of the people who are supported by the service requested flower beds, as they had previously grown their own flowers in their own gardens and for some this was no longer possible. The added benefit is that flowers can be taken home or used to brighten up the centre – all the more enjoyable in the knowledge that we have grown them ourselves. We are fortunate that we receive donations of seeds, plants, pots and fertiliser every year from two local garden centres, who are happy to support the service and this local community initiative.

The service also provides a two-course meal for everyone who attends day care on a daily basis. We do not have a cook, and a member of staff takes responsibility for producing the meal with the assistance of people with dementia. There are great benefits in being able to grow our own vegetables: we are able to take potatoes and cabbage, as well as other produce, prepare and cook it in our own kitchen and serve it for lunch. We are also able to make nutritious homemade soups and experiment with recipes we have not tried before.

Eating our own produce ensures that people who are not able to participate in maintaining the allotment can be involved in the development of menus, the preparation and cooking of meals and the serving and eating of the food prepared. Great pride is taken in eating our own produce and there are always comments on how it tastes better and how fresh and enjoyable these meals are.

The following case studies illustrate the benefits of having access to an allotment. The names of the people featured have been changed to preserve their anonymity.

Case study 1

Kate is a 74-year-old woman who was diagnosed with Alzheimer's disease four years ago. She has cared for her disabled husband, Jim, for the past 20 years. Their daughter Anne lives locally and their son James lives in England. Kate and the family are aware of her diagnosis. She began attending day care three years ago. There are other supports in place to care for Jim, including rolling respite. A key issue was the stress placed on Anne, who works full-time and has the main carer responsibility for both Mum and Dad.

Kate had benefited from a secure family childhood, living on a farm. Her father would be considered as a gentleman farmer and her mother was a housewife, running the home and caring for the children. Kate has a younger sister, Margaret, and both girls were given a good education which extended to university. Kate was encouraged to be independent and to follow her interests. She has strong socialist views and was an accomplished artist. Kate's personality demonstrated a capable, strong, independent woman who had faced many challenges in her life and overcame them successfully.

She would reflect on her childhood and younger years, explaining her enjoyment of living on the farm and being outside, taking great pleasure in observing and interacting with the nature that surrounded her. Kate also had the opportunity to travel extensively in her youth and her paintings reflected this with a focus on landscape paintings from here and abroad, visually demonstrating her love and connection to nature.

Due to her husband's illness, Kate was the person with overall responsibility in her household. She was in control, making the decisions about the running of the household, including childcare, finance, social life and interaction with external organisations and agencies.

When Kate first began attending day care she was able to speak about her frustrations and her feelings that she was losing control and unable to influence the things that were happening around her. She recognised the need for support and for her daughter to have respite from the pressure of caring for her parents. When Kate was at day care she continued to occupy a caring role, assisting with tasks, like doing the laundry, helping with meal preparation and supporting other people with dementia.

As her dementia progressed Kate became increasingly frustrated at her loss of cognitive awareness and practical abilities. She was no longer able to paint, and struggled to complete tasks like laying the table for lunch without assistance. Kate was also losing her normal inhibitions and this sometimes took the form of challenging behaviour. She was sometimes verbally aggressive or commented loudly and negatively on other people's behaviour. Day care is by its nature a group environment, and skills such as tolerance, sharing and sociability are needed. Challenging behaviour can be a demonstration that the individual is struggling to apply these skills. As individuals we all have a unique sense of our own personhood. When a person struggles to identify who they are and how others perceive them, it is important that their identity is valued and respected. This is done by offering dignity and a recognition of the person's individuality. The way to do this is to listen, and to try to decode language and behaviour. You can listen to memories of the past and transfer your understanding to the present situation.

When Kate was asked if she wished to assist with the allotment, she clearly indicated that she would like to be involved. As she began to work on the allotment, she took great satisfaction in being able to undertake and complete small tasks. She was able to identify the Latin names of trees and plants, something she had learned as a child, and was proud of her ability to teach these to others. She expressed a great appreciation of the colours, shapes, smells and sounds around her, often being able to identify things that those without an artist's eye might have missed.

As Kate's dementia progressed further, she became less and less able to communicate verbally, less able to identify the names of objects or feelings, and when feeling angry, upset, confused or frustrated would begin to sing her 'theme' tune. She was always able to remember the tune but would not always sing the correct words. This would annoy and aggravate other people within the group setting. Kate became particularly confused and disorientated when Jim was on residential respite. Although she was aware of the fact that he was on respite, her normal routine was affected. She was at home alone and because there was not the daily structure of caring for Jim, her sleep and eating patterns were disrupted, causing her to become agitated, tired and confused. It was also clear to the day care staff that Kate was experiencing some difficulty. The allotment then became a place of peace and tranquillity for her. With support from staff she was able to calm herself and re-centre. It was an opportunity to distract her and to attempt to establish how she was feeling, in an environment where she felt safe and secure and which was familiar to her.

Case study 2

Jimmy is a 78-year-old man who was diagnosed with frontal lobe dementia 18 months ago. Jimmy is aware of his diagnosis. He lives alone in a two-bedroomed ground-floor flat. Jimmy previously lived in a three-bedroomed house with his wife, who died 15 years ago. Jimmy struggled to maintain the house and moved to a smaller property, closer to his nephew, John (his only close relative). Jimmy began attending day care after being referred by John, who was concerned that Jimmy was isolated and lonely, and that spending so much time alone was causing him to become disorientated and withdrawn.

Jimmy has a lovely, easygoing personality, he loves to laugh and really enjoys company. Except for some arthritis and a slight hearing problem in his left ear, he is remarkably physically fit and he puts this down to having no vices and working in manual labour jobs his whole life. He has worked predominantly in male-orientated environments, being a milk boy in his early youth, joining the Merchant Navy and subsequently working in the Whisky Bond until he retired. It is important to all of us to be accepted and valued for the person we believe ourselves to be. Jimmy views himself as a man's man and has a positive view of himself when he is able to engage in 'masculine' activities, which is accepted by the other males in the group.

It became apparent that although Jimmy enjoys being at the centre, because of his nice nature and the gentlemanly fashion in which he conducts himself, the ladies fuss over him. He enjoys this but he is more comfortable in male company. He quickly established himself in the domino and pool league but expressed a wish to spend more time outside. He was asked if he wished to help at the allotment, and was very keen to do this.

The importance of being involved in something productive with tangible outcomes is important to Jimmy and the ability to participate in manual activities has given him a sense of well-being and has promoted his self-esteem.

Keeping healthy has always been important to Jimmy. He never smoked or drank and has always maintained a healthy diet. He has a very healthy appetite and he demonstrates a great sense of pride and self-worth when he brings potatoes and vegetables to the centre for lunch. He is very pleased when other people praise him for his efforts.

More recently, he has become less able to undertake the physical work on the allotment, but he has been encouraged to undertake less physical but equally important tasks, such as potting seedlings and re-potting other plants. Jimmy also enters into animated and engaging conversations with the gentleman who works the allotment next door, and thereby gains valuable confidence from having his knowledge and skills acknowledged.

There is an added thread to Jimmy's working on the allotment. His nephew John is one of our volunteers and he supports and assists people with dementia who work on the allotment. John is Jimmy's main carer and has the stresses and worries that go along with caring for an older relative with dementia. This changes family relationships. John has fond memories of his uncle when he was younger and has always seen him as an excellent role model, who was attentive to his nephew and spent quality time with him. This aspect of their relationship had been lost. However, working on the allotment together gave them both the opportunity to enjoy an activity in a quiet, tranquil environment with none of the pressures felt when dealing with day-to-day issues, like making sure the household bills are paid and the laundry is done. John learned that he could spend time with his uncle that did not feel stressful and that he considered to be quality time.

Although there are some problems with the allotment, which in our case include access issues, seasonal workload variables and the Scottish weather, there are also many positive benefits for the people with dementia. Within the wider society, working with volunteers and having contact with other people who also have allotments contributes to raising awareness and reducing stigma.

Creating a therapeutic environment incorporating nature into a care setting has several benefits for individuals, which include enhanced cognition, psychological and physical well-being, and improved behaviour. The physical benefits include helping to keep limbs and joints supple and functional, and contribute to reducing the risks of heart disease, diabetes and obesity. Eating the produce grown on the allotment also contributes towards a healthy, balanced diet and being able to prepare nutritious meals. It also encourages physical activity, even amongst the less physically able, and invites social interaction on a one-to-one basis and within a group.

The mental and spiritual benefits include the opportunity to escape to a tranquil space, in a world where there is constant noise and everyone and everything is busy. There is a real benefit to being able to do your own thing in a place that is peaceful and not overstimulating to the senses.

Working on an allotment can help with life skills and can provide a sense of achievement, satisfaction and pride (see Figure 10.2). It is an empowering experience that can build self-esteem and relieve stress.

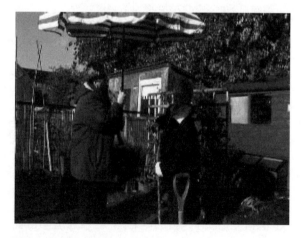

Figure 10.2 Working on an allotment can provide a sense of achievement, satisfaction and pride
Photo: Lorraine Robertson

Visually, a well cared-for and maintained allotment is aesthetically pleasing and contributes towards the sense of peace, tranquillity and well-being. Allotments are often associated with the romance of being in contact with the land and can remind people of a time when hard work was important, and supporting your family and contributing to your community were strongly-held values. Working on an allotment offers people the opportunity to be creative and productive.

Conversations on next year's planting, how the current crops are coming along, and sharing knowledge, skills and tips that have sometimes been passed down through generations, are valuable in maintaining communication and interpersonal skills. Being able to reminisce about personal experiences of working on farms, allotments or the vegetable plot in the back garden makes a valuable contribution to cognitive awareness and the person's sense of self-worth.

An allotment is a beneficial resource to any service supporting those with dementia in their local community.

Things Aren't What They Used to Be[1]

TREVOR JARVIS

Things aren't what they used to be
Can't remember when to plant them plants
Sow them seeds, I don't know when to sow
Can't remember when
Things aren't what they used to be
Is it today when I mow or do I sow, I don't know?
Can't remember when
Things aren't what they used to be
Did I hoe or did I sow, I don't know
Can't remember when
Things aren't what they used to be
Did I water them plants or did I sow or do I mow,
I don't know where to go, or what to sow
Can't remember when
Things aren't what they used to be
Things aren't what they used to be
Can't remember when
Can't remember when
Just can't remember.

---

1   To be sung to the tune of 'Fings ain't wot they used to be'.

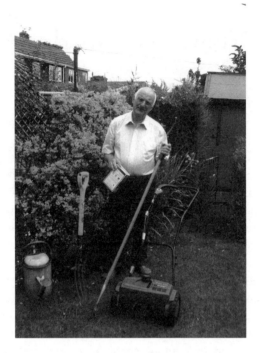

Trevor in his garden – 'a garden that holds all my memories'
Photo: Ann Jarvis

Chapter 11

Creativity Outdoors

CLAIRE CRAIG

Outside space is: freedom, fresh air, fun, fiesta, play, peacefulness, contemplation, restoration, picnics, adventure, discovery, growth, change, barbecues, seasons, sunshine, love, raindrops.

A few years ago after a visit to Barcelona and inspired by Gaudi, we decided to transform our back yard into an artists' garden. Rather than sticking to the usual browns and greens previously used to paint the fence, we took a bold approach – bright blues, vibrant yellows and reds. A mosaic made from recycled tiles and broken crockery adorned the garage wall and coloured gravels the floor. It was transformed overnight. We were very pleased with ourselves and wanting to show this off, invited friends and neighbours to a grand unveiling with a barbecue. Naturally conversation turned to outdoor space in general and we were both excited and surprised to hear our neighbours tell of their own creations. A very good friend of ours, an esteemed professor, shared that he had transformed his back garden into a model railway village complete with stations and train-tracks. 'For a long time I pretended that it was for the children,' he confided, 'but in truth they left home over a decade ago. The space became my haven, you see.' Another friend described how she had turned a shed into a beach hut. 'In our youth we had such good memories of sitting on the seafront at Scarborough that when both of us became ill and could no longer travel we decided to bring a corner of Scarborough to Barnsley. Even now he'll look at me and say, 'Hilda, are you going to make a flask up?' and we'll sit at the bottom of the garden in our deckchairs, listening to the radio and imagining that we can smell the sea.'

Outdoor spaces present many possibilities for creative ventures. On one level, outdoors can be a place to *express* creativity. Gardening and garden design are extremely creative acts promoting expression through the choosing and placing of various plants and shrubs, in deciding colour and scent combinations or the theme of the garden (vegetable, flower, kitchen, herb). When people move into new environments, outdoor spaces can offer a sense of continuity and orientation and help people to feel 'grounded'. This space may be a place to exhibit works of art, sculptures, mosaic and paintings, or act as the backdrop to drama and performance.

The outdoors can also *inspire* creativity, offering themes or subjects for painting, photography or writing. Significantly, because outdoor spaces operate within a different set of parameters to indoor spaces, activities that might be deemed too 'messy' and unacceptable for indoors (usually those involving paint or dirt and water) are suddenly deemed appropriate and acceptable outside, permitting people to move beyond the sterile environment, gain the most from the sensory component of the materials and literally 'get their hands dirty'. This chapter begins with a brief consideration of the benefits of nature and outside spaces before looking at the opportunities for creativity that they offer people in terms of expressing and inspiring creativity.

As a starting point I would like to invite you to reflect for a few moments on your relationship with nature and the ways you may use outdoor space. Try the following exercise:

- Do you have a garden or a patio? If so, what does it say about you? Does the space reflect anything of your personality?

- Look through a photograph album. Make a note of how many of the images in your album are of outdoor spaces. How do you feel when you look at these images?

- Have you ever been inspired to paint or draw the landscape or write about it?

- Our view of outdoor space changes as time passes. How have you used space at different periods of your life? For instance, when you were younger the outdoors may have been associated with play; in your teens it might have been about love, romance, courtship; at the moment you may associate outdoors as being about hard work (growing things), or about entertaining, or about self-expression and identity.

So why the outdoors? There is a growing body of evidence to suggest that there is a strong relationship between nature, the outdoors, health and well-being. First, it will come as no surprise that increasing activity levels by spending time outdoors can result in a number of physical benefits (Haennel and Lemire 2002). Being physically engaged in outdoor activities can lead to increased appetite, improved sleep pattern and changes in stamina (Chalfont 2007).

There is much to be said about context here. Frequently I am privy to conversations in the care home trying to persuade residents to take part in chair exercises. It is interesting that individuals who refuse point blank to participate in these indoor physical pursuits will happily bend, stretch and move around outdoors when engaging in simple gardening tasks they find meaningful, providing the opportunity to channel energies and experience feelings of 'productiveness'.

However, the benefits are not confined to physical health. Care environments can be noisy and confusing places, so perhaps it is also not surprising that a study of nursing home residents by Rappe, Kivela and Rita (2006) found that spending time outdoors led to improved perceptions of health and well-being. Other studies have shown there to be a positive relationship between walking and communication for people with dementia (Cott *et al.* 2002; Friedman and Tappen 1991); and the literature is unanimous regarding the overall positive impact of being outdoors on well-being (Duggan, Blackman, Martyr and Van Schaik 2008). Duggan *et al.* conclude that 'maintaining outdoor activity is likely to be an effective preventative measure in extending the period of good quality living…it should therefore be considered in planning for both residential care and community living in the future' (p.191).

Yet, in spite of these known benefits, the importance of outdoor space is frequently overlooked during the design of many environments where people with dementia live. As a consequence the rooms or the 'wing' allocated to people diagnosed with dementia are often situated on the second or third floor of a complex, making independent access to the outside virtually impossible. For individuals living in ground-floor accommodation, inviting outdoor spaces may be rendered inaccessible by locked patio doors or steep concrete steps and nasty metal door jambs. Attitudes can be just as restrictive. During a recent visit to a care home my suggestion to visit the local botanical gardens for a walk was met with the unanimous, genuine and concerned response, 'How can you expect people to walk? It's not even summer, haven't you heard of pneumonia?' One person said accusingly, 'If someone dies it will be your fault!' With such strongly held pre-conceptions it is perhaps unsurprising that people with dementia are so often denied the opportunity to physically go outdoors.

Clearly there are many deeply held beliefs to challenge. In my experience, however, exploring the *creative potential* of outdoor spaces can go some way towards providing a reason or an opportunity for people to access the outside, that is felt to be acceptable to staff. Here are some examples from my own work.

One of the most effective approaches is to reduce the division of 'outside' and 'inside' space so the outdoors becomes a natural extension of the inner space. Creating outdoor galleries to display art work provides an excellent mechanism for this and offers people with dementia and their families a reason to spend time together outside. This has the further advantage of creating additional space, which is so important in many settings where space is so often at a premium.

Using garden or patio areas to display or frame pieces of art that have been created provides a different feel to the work, as well as offering an outdoor gallery which people with dementia, staff and carers can enjoy. Naturally, some materials lend themselves more easily to surviving the outdoor elements: ceramics, mosaic and wooden structures do very well and are made for outside. However, with a little imagination it is possible to introduce other art forms into these spaces. For example, poetry and imagery can be written or painted on stones. When varnished these pieces can add interest to an environment and form the basis of poetry walks and storytelling. Photographs and pieces of art can be protected from the elements if they are displayed in clear perspex containers, bottles or jars.

Another way to support this approach is to invite people to put their creative mark on the outdoor space. People with dementia often live in environments where they have very little control over the space they inhabit. Room size and health and safety requirements can make even the simplest of 'home touches' difficult to introduce. Outside spaces, therefore, can offer new and exciting possibilities for individuals to extend their living space by putting their own creative mark on the environment.

Individuals can be invited to 'design' their own patch of land. This might be in relation to a colour scheme, or based around a theme. For example, in a care home I have recently been working in, one person has designated a small piece of the patio area as 'her patch'. Having spent much of her early life living in Egypt, she created a 'corner of the Sahara' complete with sand and rocks. On a sunny day she sits in a deckchair with her back to the home, her shoes and socks cast to one side, and her feet in the sand. It is a wonderful sight to behold. Another person in the same home has created a 'remembrance garden' – each plant, bought by a member of his family, has a particular association. Family members have used metal labels to write short descriptions... 'Do you remember when you mowed over the lavender in the front garden, Dad?' 'Do you remember the sage that turned out to be catmint?' It is a really beautiful place to be, full of positive associations and memories.

Other themes that could be explored include the following:

- *Mood*: a garden to reflect moods.

- *Geography*: garden areas themed around different parts of the world.

- *Colour*: outdoor spaces with an emphasis on a particular colour.

- *Landscape*: whether this is the seaside or a natural meadow.

Small, flagged areas can present just as many possibilities, and I have worked in homes where we have decorated paving slabs with mosaic or paint. Once, as part of a 'Film Festival evening', residents made hand prints in the same way as stars do on the Hollywood Boulevard, but rather than being in concrete, these were made in chalk. If this is difficult, individually painted or themed planters can be just as meaningful. People with dementia have decorated both the outside and inside of these, either through painting or by using mosaic tiles before selecting the plants and creating individual planting schemes. I have learned much about the person through this process, particularly in relation to an individual's capacity for humour and fun. For instance, Bob, a person with dementia, named his creation 'Lost the pot' and Eric, who decorated his planter with brightly coloured circles, named it 'Spot the pot'.

Indoor arts-based sessions can be dedicated to planning and designing these spaces, whether this is creating a pre-design using collage, paint or another media, or creating concept maps for ideas. You may decide to use the outside space as an opportunity to work with the wider community, inviting students from local horticultural or arts colleges to share their ideas. This can create a sense of community connectedness. I am aware of a project in my locality where young people from the secondary school are working with people in one care environment to create a 'recycled' garden, looking at ways of using things that might otherwise be thrown away. Many of the older people are of the generation of 'make do and mend' and are offering invaluable ideas about ways to use and re-use objects, and in return the young people are helping with the physical construction of the space.

So far I have described ways that outdoors can offer opportunity to *express* creativity, breaking down the division between indoors and outdoors. I would now like to consider the potential of the outdoors to *inspire* creativity.

For centuries, outdoor spaces have been the inspiration for art and creativity. Go to any gallery and reflect on how many paintings represent some facet of nature: rolling landscapes, gardens, seascapes, dramatic sunrises and sunsets. Similarly think of the number of poems inspired by the outdoors – Wordsworth's 'Daffodils'; Arnold's 'Dover Beach'; Keats' 'Ode to a Nightingale'. I enjoy inviting people with dementia to engage in creative activities in outdoor spaces, whether this is painting and drawing, writing poetry or taking photographs.

Engaging in creative activities outdoors offers a very different experience to doing the same activity inside. I have spent a great deal of time trying to untangle why this might be so. For one thing, there are fewer physical constraints, and as a facilitator I am sure that because of this I am naturally more relaxed and any anxiety I might project dissipates.

Just being outdoors can also be much quieter, feel more peaceful. Many of the hospital and care home environments I visit, by their nature can be noisy and feel chaotic, alarm bells ringing, staff rushing to complete tasks. Just being outside, away from the daily hustle and bustle, offers an opportunity for peace and quiet, making it easier to concentrate.

I am frequently struck by the improvements in the quality of people's speech and ability to engage in activity when outdoors. In part, I am sure that this is because of the space that being outside offers. Jacqueline, a person with dementia, when stepping outdoors into the fresh air, sighed and said in a very matter-of-fact tone, 'Now we can think,' which again made me reflect on how the outdoors is as much about offering mental space as it is about the physical. Another person with dementia, Joan, following a painting activity, looked at me directly and said, 'This is real.'

Perhaps one of the greatest ironies is that many of the places where people with dementia live and are cared for are in artificially constructed environments – two-dimensional shadows of reality where light, temperature, atmosphere are completely regulated. As a consequence, when creative activities take place outdoors, the experience becomes three-dimensional and the sensory component contributes as much to the quality of the end-product as to the process of engagement.

Clearly these opportunities are not confined to people with dementia living in care environments. A person I recently visited at home who has just received a diagnosis of dementia was in the back garden, up to his elbows in mud. 'It helps me feel connected,' he said. 'Out here I have a purpose. I worry about losing my confidence.'

This issue of confidence is one that has arisen frequently in my discussions with people with dementia, both in their own homes and in care homes, particularly if someone has spent a great deal of time indoors or is fearful of becoming lost. Again, shared activities outdoors can offer a focus and help people to maintain and build confidence, whether living at home or in care environments.

Photography is something that lends itself particularly well to this. The idea of 'taking a camera for a walk' can provide a reason to go outside and offer purpose. 'Captured Memories' is an example of one such project that took place in Stirling. People with dementia were invited to record their experiences of community outings, using disposable cameras. Rosas Mitchell, facilitator of the project, describes some of the benefits as follows:

- Group members' sense of self and identity were affirmed, enabling individuals to talk about their life story in relation to what they had seen and photographed.

- Self-esteem and sense of value increased by developing skills.

- People were able to communicate better with each other.

(Mitchell 2005)

Feedback from people with dementia was very positive. One person said, 'It was the best day I had had for a very long time.' Significantly, group members commented on the experience of being in nature: 'I like that forest thing,' and 'The greenery reminded me of the area where I was growing up. It was on a farm and we used to have guests to stay' (Mitchell 2005, pp.20–21). The comments are a poignant reminder that nature and outside space are part of our inner landscapes, our life experiences (see Figure 11.1).

Many activities are linked to specific seasons of the year, marking the passage of time. Again, I like to use creative activities to tap into these. Harvest festivals, carol singing, Easter-egg hunts are ways of engaging with the outside, helping to orientate people to the passage of time. Such events can be extremely sociable. In the city of Sheffield where I work we have the Care Home Olympics, where residents from different care homes compete in outdoor games, building a sense of community and offering an opportunity for social interaction. Outdoor picnics, barbecues and fiestas, focus on the social element of food and eating and offer opportunities to engage with the wider community. In one district with a large Chinese population the care home is invited to share in their festivities and take part in the 'Festival of Light', releasing hundreds of Chinese paper lanterns, lovingly made by residents, into the evening sky.

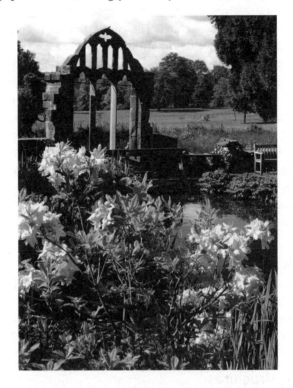

Figure 11.1 Nature and outside space are part of our inner landscapes, our life experiences
Photo: Claire Craig

The outdoors also offers opportunities for music and drama. The smallest area of grass can offer a perfect backdrop for performances and opportunities for celebration. For instance, individuals may wish to share their work created during poetry sessions, or to perform short scripts. Local drama societies may appreciate the opportunity to rehearse their productions, and you could invite bands or choirs to share well-known medleys. I have visited care homes that have used this as an opportunity to raise money – the combination of strawberry teas and music outdoors have met with great success.

You can also link the outside space with other, more sombre life rhythms – a remembrance garden, for example, where people's lives can be celebrated by the simple act of tying a ribbon on a tree or placing a decorated stone in a sacred space.

Clearly, when engaging in creative activities outdoors there are things to consider. Dress, for one, is very important. Good footwear and appropriate clothing are essential. The contrast in temperature between indoors and outdoors can be dramatic and an extra jumper or blanket can make the experience of sitting for a length of time more pleasant. If sessions are taking place in summer some form of skin protection is required. A garden umbrella may offer shade and sun-screen can block out the ultraviolet rays that damage the skin. If you are going to engage in painting or claywork, make sure that you provide tables or easels, and chairs for people to rest on. It is also important to remember that if a person hasn't been outside for some time they may initially lack confidence.

Here are some ideas for ways of using outside space as the starting point for activities.

Creative writing

Sitting outside, sharing a view with someone, listening to what they say and capturing these words in written form can be extremely validating for the person and can also enable you to pause for a second, to listen and reflect on what someone is communicating.

Creating structures

The easiest structures comprise single words or word lists; you might, for instance, ask someone to look around them and think of words to describe:

- a favourite view
- a special place
- a time of day.

Here is an example of a list of words spoken by an older person to describe a special place:

'Warm breeze, honeysuckle, a red rose, a shaded spot, a secret kiss, at peace, loved.'

Found objects

Outside spaces offer opportunities for exploration. One activity that works very well is to invite the person to seek out objects that can then act as stimuli for writing. These objects and textures often carry strong associations which can stimulate the imagination. Once an object has been identified, allow the person space and time to explore it through touch. Sometimes I have invited the person to imagine how the object could be used, or to picture who might have used it in the past or how it came to be outdoors. It is amazing the types of objects that have been 'discovered' outdoors, including keys, coins, gardening gloves and a whistle!

Engaging the senses

Nature offers the opportunity to engage in a sensory experience. This sensory component can also offer a structure for writing. When sharing this with someone I tend to take an A4 sheet of paper and divide it into six squares, as this can offer a visual prompt. In five of the squares I write down one of the senses (substituting temperature for taste) and in the sixth square I write down the word 'feeling'. Then, sitting with the person, we identify together the scents and aromas, textures, sounds, sights, etc., recording these in each of the boxes – and finally how the person feels. Such is the power of this activity in terms of tapping into memories that we rarely get beyond the first two. The words can then form the basis of creative writing or a relaxation exercise, enabling the person to connect to nature even when they are physically indoors.

Conclusion

I have offered just a few examples here about the opportunities that outside spaces offer in relation to creativity and self-expression. The outdoors provides context for many of the activities we engage in, which in turn reflect facets of our personality and make us who we are. To deny a person this is to deny them a huge part of their life. It seems apt, given that creativity is about growth and adventure, that it should offer a reason and a way to access this space and in doing so to access activities:

> [that] are a part of older people's lives, enable them to participate and contribute, preserve personal identity and sense of self, afford ongoing meaningful roles within the communal setting and make a place feel less institutional and more like home. (Chalfont 2007, p.25)

References

Chalfont, G. (2007) 'The dementia care garden: Part of daily life and activity.' *Journal of Dementia Care*, November/December, 24–28.

Cott, C.A., Dawson, P., Sidani, S. and Wells, D. (2002) 'The effects of a walking/talking program on communication, ambulation, and functional status in residents with Alzheimer disease.' *Alzheimer Disease and Associated Disorders 16*, 2, 81–87.

Duggan, S., Blackman, T., Martyr, A. and Van Schaik, P. (2008) 'The impact of early dementia on outdoor life: "A shrinking world?"' *Dementia 7*, 191–204.

Friedman, R. and Tappen, R.M. (1991) 'The effect of planned walking on communication in Alzheimer's disease.' *Journal of the American Geriatrics Society 40*, 650–654.

Haennel, R.G. and Lemire, F. (2002) 'Physical activity to prevent cardiovascular disease: How much is enough?' *Canadian Family Physician 48*, 65–71.

Mitchell, R. (2005) 'Captured Memories.' A Photography project in a Drop-In Centre. Stirling: Dementia Services Development Centre.

Rappe, E., Kivela, S.L. and Rita, H. (2006) 'Visiting outdoor green environments positively impacts self-rated health among older people in long-term care.' *Horttechnology 16*, 1, 55–59.

Chapter 12

The Therapeutic
MOUNTAIN

The AlzheimUr CENTRE
(Murcia, Spain)

HALLDÓRA ARNARDÓTTIR AND JAVIER SÁNCHEZ MERINA

In the design of the AlzheimUr CENTRE in the hills of Montecantalar in Murcia, nature and the mountain have played a leading role in our aim to achieve therapeutic architecture.

The site was donated to the AlzheimUr Foundation in 2006 by the town council to accommodate the dementia unit at the Hospital Virgen de la Arrixaca (which serves the region of Murcia) and laboratories with a brain bank, as well as a day centre and a family training centre. The neurologist and head of the unit, Carmen Antúnez, had come up with the vision of these four core zones. Uniting these different aspects together in one place was a completely new concept in Spain.

As a consequence of the aging population, dementia is increasingly being diagnosed in the east Spanish region of Murcia; currently close to 10,000 people. This growing group is vulnerable and in need of integrated, value-based medicine. They generate great interest and concern, not least because their care results in immense expense for the health and social care system.

Within this context of improving the life of the people with dementia and their families, the AlzheimUr CENTRE builds on values to create an environment emphasising understanding rather than change. It bases its architectural language on the social culture directly linked with the climate and ways of living, an approach that is in itself a non-pharmacologic therapy.

Located in the south-east of Spain, between the regions of Andalusia, Castilla, La Mancha and Valencia, the region of Murcia is known for its acres of orchards and vegetable fields through which the Segura River runs. Even the great expanse of the municipal area is made up of different landscapes: extensive tracks of heavily eroded uncultivated land with little vegetation, groves of Carrasco pine trees in the mountain ranges close to the coast, and flat valleys.

Before starting the design process, the first meeting of the design team was at the mountain Montecantalar to get familiar with its paths and qualities: fragrances, colours, sounds and light.

The paths, grown into the hills, seemed to have kept their own memories from bringing together families and groups of friends for going on picnics. As we climbed up the hill, we perceived the different densities of vegetation that produced subtle variations in light and views, aromas and sounds. There were multiple sensory elements like the scent of orange blossom, thyme and rosemary; the rhythmical sound of the cicada, and bird songs; greenish light and fresh shadows, as we walked from cultivated orchards at the bottom of the mountain, through pine trees to a rocky and open landscape at the top. Different atmospheres appeared throughout the route, from open and luminous surroundings to a much more intimate ambience filtered by extraordinary qualities of light.

A labyrinth of pine trunks created dense shadows as if it were a web of parasols. Further on, an irrigation ditch appeared, and again the air became dry. This made us think of ways to collect and conserve water. As we reached the peak, the slope became sharper and the uniqueness of the site more visible.

Back in the office, the first task was to set up a weblog, www.alzheimurcentre.blogspot.com, to document our working process and as a tool for exchanging ideas on the internet around the world. The next step was to draw an elevation of the mountain's qualities, and we also made a large, scale model of the mountain. Working with both techniques helped us to get a sense of different layers and paths that could serve as connection points and reinforce the building's relationship with the qualities of the mountain. Essentially, they were studies of spatial concepts and joints, the various levels in the hill that corresponded with the cultivated orchards, pine trees and rocks, and how these levels could join the building's structure.

The shape of the landscape was extremely powerful in the search for an equilibrium that the design of the AlzheimUr CENTRE wanted to achieve. From the vantage point of the top of the mountain, one could see how the paths met to embrace the mountain. Working physically with the model and critically evaluating each decision, the mountain became accommodated. The pavilions appeared, gently taking their place along the paths: two day centres, laboratories and brain banks, the dementia unit, the family training centre, the offices, the theatre and the cafeteria. Together, they constitute a building complex that joins the mountain, maintaining its trees and making use of its orientation and views. The centre as a whole adapted itself to the mountain and the pavilions were made to fit, to the point that they almost become the mountain (see Figures 12.1 and 12.2).

As the design process evolved, we realised how rich in complexities and possibilities the centre was becoming. Apart from its role for day care and a research centre, the building also stimulates studies of the disease, which embrace aspects of the general culture and the performing arts. Besides establishing connections with nature and the soil, following the paths on the mountain is reminiscent of a number of characteristics of the city for the users; of finding and sharing things during walks. The good climate of the Mediterranean encourages people to enjoy social life in the squares. In so doing they organise and discover activities such as lectures, informal talks, cinema, music and dance, exhibitions and workshops.

Situated along one of the paths, the auditorium is a 'found-object' like a *town square* in the city, a place one can both pass through and/or go to. Here culture is fostered, communication encouraged, and knowledge and technology are on display. The town square is a heterogeneous open place, it welcomes changes and is, in that sense, optimistic. It is full of possibilities. Going to the theatre and summer cinema stimulates memories. It is *food for thought* with the added ingredient of the indispensable sandwich with *jamón* (cured ham) and a drink. This is no different from years before during the warm summer nights, when the same people – then young – went to watch a film which was interrupted by the sound of crickets, and where the walls of the cinema were covered with impressive bougainvilleas climbing up until they seemed to merge with the sky. They are memories that cannot be forgotten.

Remembering things past in the context of Murcia, more memories than the folk traditions or the blue of the Mediterranean Sea come to mind. The fragrance of the *azahar* (orange flower) fills the air, the orange sunlight embraces the mountains in the afternoons, the hot breeze strokes your cheeks in the summer nights, the peculiar grey colour and texture of the olive tree, the different patios offering shade as the day goes by, the people taking their chairs into the street in order to converse with their neighbours – all reach deep into the memory.

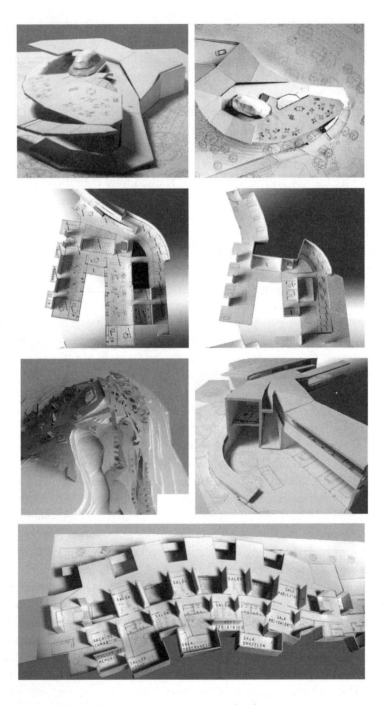

Figure 12.1 The plan for the AlzheimUr CENTRE takes shape
Photos: Copyright © SARQ Architecture Office

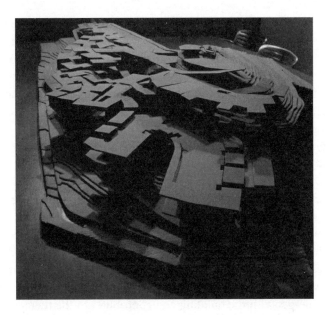

Figure 12.2 Architect's model for the AlzheimUr CENTRE
Photo: Copyright © SARQ Architecture Office

In our culture, there are a number of activities that draw people up to a mountain. On the day of '*la mona*' (special rolls normally served with a hard boiled egg), people go to the slopes of the mountains with families and groups of friends to enjoy a day out together in nature, having rice with rabbit, salads, omelettes, raw broad beans, '*las monas*' and other foods particular to Easter.

Another tradition is the feeling the general public has for the patron saint who protects the city of Murcia: Virgin Fuensanta. This saint resides in the sanctuary in the mountain, known as Hondoyuelo. The history of how Fuensanta became the protector of the city emphasises the importance of water in the region. At the time the Virgin was first taken down from the sanctuary and into the city on 17 January 1694, it had been extremely dry for months. The farmers desperately needed rain. In this religious procession, the Virgin's followers begged her for rain. At the end of long prayers, it rained heavily, which even ended in snow. At that time, the protector of Murcia was Virgin Santa María de la Arrixaca – but her popularity started to decline due to the recurring miracles of water during the subsequent religious processions of Fuensanta, which made her, in the year 1731, the new patron saint for Murcia and the city's orchards.

Water is obviously an important subject in Murcia. The region is one of the driest in Spain as it has, on average, more than 300 days of sun per year and rainfall is irregular. Occasionally Murcia has heavy rains, when the precipitation for the entire year will fall over the course of a few days. The design of the centre was adapted to this reality and rainwater is collected in underground tanks. This water is then used to water the plants on the site.

The different roof terraces are planted with local vegetation (thyme, rosemary, etc.) that provides humidity to the atmosphere, as well as insulation for the roof. The constant fragrance reinforces the connection with the mountain inherent in the vegetation. Capturing the mountain's overlapping aromas, the roofs of the different pavilions become terraces where plants fill the air with their fragrance. In that way, the vegetation of the orchards seem to climb up the levels of the building to the different terraces accessible to the people with dementia, where they can participate in workshops and non-pharmacological treatment. In that sense, Murcia's orchard merges with the building and contributes to the therapies.

The mountain is a constant landmark and a reference for orientation for the people with dementia. Walking to the different pavilions, they and other users of the building sense how the activities are organised along the mountain, as the view towards the orchard and horizon open on to the other side. The relationship between the topography of the land and the trees determined the spaces of the pavilions. We drew a grid of the existing vegetation and calculated the height from the ground to the top of the trees to find out the space under the canopy. In this way we established different planes that enabled the building to intertwine with the vegetation.

In principle, the maximum difference in levels between any two connecting points is no more than four metres, and the slope no more than 6 per cent, so as to connect different parts of the construction in a comfortable way for the users and to respect the land. Open patios and closed spaces knit into the mountain, creating shade and natural cross-ventilation, which is refreshing; a fundamental element for a climate such as that of Murcia. The open patios with trees and evergreen plants are drawn from the Arab tradition of domestic houses to achieve a fresh atmosphere in the interior spaces. Furthermore, it brings people closer to nature and the notion of time.

This search for equilibrium between the mountain, nature and the building for the benefit of the people with dementia is tightly bound to the complex range of colours and colour contrasts. Contextual factors of perception and light make colours interact, creating harmony, or disharmony, depending on how they are juxtaposed. In AlzheimUr CENTRE the building materials include natural wood, stones and plants, whose colours play a part in recalling memories of picking olives, reading the newspaper or a book under a grapevine, or strolling in an orange orchard and picking a fruit for refreshment. The colours are not merely part of nature but help to recall living culture and nurture the inner self of the people with dementia.

As a way of presenting *a day in the AlzheimUr CENTRE*, at the ceremony of laying the foundation stone all these values were drawn together in a video where a person with dementia described her feelings and preoccupations – 'Creating Memories'. This video setting drew a picture of the future, of how we desire the centre to be used or experienced when the building process was finished.

> Today I turn 70. I am an Alzheimer patient and, although you won't believe it, today I live only from my memories.
>
> For the past few years, I have kept making efforts in remembering things…
>
> In the mornings, the orchards come back to my mind. The murmuring of the water and the fragrance of lemon blossoms accompany me as I water the fruit trees and pick the lemons. I then take some breaths… I sit down in the shade, and again, I imagine myself drawing with the colours of the bougainvilleas – something that has always relaxed me.
>
> Finally, the sound of the cicada signals time for lunch, and the sky turns into sparkles from the sun. Rice and rabbit with big snails: my speciality.
>
> Later, I play ludo with a group of friends while we digest our lunch. The men like dominos a lot…but '*mus*' (a Spanish card game) even more.
>
> Other days, I like simply sitting on the patio and to chat, or sitting in the shade under the trees. Again, time passes very slowly. I go back in my memory – it's like not having to wait for the day of '*la monà*' to go up the mountain.
>
> From there, I enjoyed the views on to Murcia's orchards: breeze with a tablecloth square, red afternoon light and birds. An afternoon lengthening into the night.
>
> Often, during rainy days, I look towards the mountains. The drops fall slowly from the needles of the pine trees.

Am I dreaming or am I already awake? … What happened just a short time ago reappears with apparent clarity. This is because all my memories originate from AlzheimUr CENTRE.

Every time I enter the CENTRE I find fragments of myself, linked to my story. When we are young, we never aim to create memories… They happen spontaneously, we are preoccupied with living.

At this stage, you are eager to find a way of holding onto and keeping the memory of things. Fortunately, this can also be built. I feel it every morning at breakfast, during my walks… dancing, and in the orchard fields.

Inside my old mountain that now makes an effort to embody memories.

In the AlzheimUr CENTRE, the architecture has learnt from the mountain and respects its pathways that evoke emotions and surprises, fragrances, breezes, variations of light, views, hidden stories and memories, orientations, shadows, freshness, sounds and topographies. Each of these elements is an essential part of this architecture, where the pine tree is just as important a building material as concrete or steel, in constructing a therapeutic mountain.

Chapter 13

Three Voices

SCOTTISH DEMENTIA WORKING GROUP

1. Ross Campbell

I worked on a farm when I was younger and that was where my love of outdoor spaces started. My hobbies were shooting and fishing – both outdoor activities, and I found them totally relaxing. I've had to give up shooting but I still go fishing – I often go out in a boat and I love the wide open spaces. I also walk the dog every day, anywhere from four to eight miles. I find it peaceful and I get to meet other dog walkers and we talk about the countryside. Being outdoors takes my tempo down and I go home fully refreshed. If I feel stressed when I go out, I come home feeling fine. I describe the outdoors as 'nature within nature itself'.

2. Nancy McAdam

I live in a croft on the Black Isle – I describe it as the 'end of the world'. I live my life outdoors – almost all of the time I am outside and I find it fantastic. When my house was busy with visitors, I even slept in the garden in a yurt. I grow lots of veggies and fruit and I am always planning ahead with what to sow next. My life is having my hands in the soil.

3. Agnes Houston

If I am feeling stressed I take myself off for a good brisk walk and I always feel better afterwards, ready to face the world again. I live in a town but I built myself a secret garden. I did my *t'ai chi* there every morning and I would eat my porridge there. I thought I couldn't be seen, but a neighbour spotted me from an upstairs window. She told my daughter that she thought I had flipped! I love to touch nature and be back to nature. It is like being reborn, it gets rid of the stress and I feel light.

Also, my brother-in-law is in the end stage of dementia. I visited him in his nursing home. The nurse took his bed to an open window so that he could feel the breeze and he gave a deep sigh of satisfaction, like when you have just eaten a really good meal.

Chapter 14

Arne Naess

A Reflection

PETER WHITEHOUSE

Most people think the world is divided into two groups of people, those with Alzheimer's and those afraid of getting it. Or to put it another way, they believe that human beings can be classified into people with dementia, their caregivers, and the rest of us on the planet. For me Arne Naess, the inspiring Norwegian philosopher, single-handedly puts a corrective lens on those distortions.

As the youngest full professor ever at the University of Oslo, Arne included academic buildings on the list of mountains and other high structures he scaled – in this case because he allegedly would lose the keys to his office. He was a serious and vigorous amateur mountaineer who lived part of the year in his much beloved Tvergastein (T) hut on the Hardangervidda mountain plateau, after which he named his personal philosophy, Ecosophy T. He invented the concept of deep ecology to help human beings appreciate their profound practical and spiritual connections to nature. He borrowed from Aldo Leopold the expression that we must learn to 'think like a mountain', to ask us to focus on long-range, broad-based, inspiring, humble, and sustainable ways of understanding the world. He left his academic post and became an environmental activist inspired by Gandhi's nonviolent methods and worked at times with the Green Party. At one time he chained himself to equipment to block the development of a dam.

The last time I saw Arne I brought him several months' supply of Horlicks, a British powdered malted milk drink that was his favorite. When I first met Arne on top of a mountain (in a restaurant) above Oslo I already knew he had dementia, although he was living at home. Kit-Fai, his devoted Chinese wife, needed to tie his shoelaces. The next time I visited him he was in a nursing home. He died a few months later in 2009 at the age of 97.

Arne was so full of joyful life and great stories. Even when his short-term memory had almost completely failed, he could communicate his love of nature and even use his long-term memory to discuss his philosophy and share stories. When I visited Arne, I had just spent a week taking the Hurtigruten coastal liner from Trondheim to Tromso above the Arctic Circle. I was there on May 17, National Constitution Day, and attended parades with many splendid national costumes. I felt the spirit of Norway that Arne also emanated. Many people told me (including those in the Alzheimer's Association) that Arne was an inspiration to the whole country (and beyond, I might add) – this despite his dementia.

So Arne was a person with a quite profound dementia who also demonstrated care towards not only his wife and me but also the whole planet. Many people with dementia are touring the world adding their voices to the discussion about reframing dementia. They are, of course, not typical, because most people with dementia cannot maintain the kind of busy writing and speaking schedules of these international stars. Arne was a deep thinker of global scope. He was a person with dementia who inspired even in a state of rather profound dementia.

As a person with Celtic roots from a clan based in Scotland, I always felt a deep resonance with nature based in that indigenous spiritual tradition. I have spent much time climbing mountains in Scotland, particularly the mystical Eildon Hills near Melrose, said to be the home of the ghosts of both King Arthur and the Faerie Queen. When visiting the northernmost Orkney Islands I had the sense that I must have had some of Arne's Norwegian blood in me (if not literally then figuratively, although those Vikings did visit many of the places my family lived). It is ironic that my Scottish family was in merchant shipping, just as Arne's family was. Arne Naess Junior, the philosopher's nephew, worked with my godfather, and Arne Jr gave a surprise address at my uncle's retirement. That part of the family had the surname Denholm – a name of Scandinavian origin. Hence I am now ready to claim a deep (perhaps even DNA) connection to the Naess family. Arne Jr actually married Diana Ross, the famous African-American singer, but tragically he was killed in a mountaineering accident.

The thinking and humility of deep ecology should tell us all that we have cognitive limitations in understanding ecosystems and challenges to our stewardship for nature. We are all impaired in our activities of living, like failing to eat healthy food and dispose properly of our 'waste'. The wisdom of Arne Naess with dementia is more profound for me than much of the knowledge of so-called Alzheimer's experts. We are coming to recognise that we are all at risk of dementia, and we all live in a continuum of cognitive aging. We should all be carers of each other. The label 'Alzheimer's' given to one person should not result in assigning another the appellation 'caregiver', somehow potentially robbing the person with dementia from giving care to others as well. So-called 'Alzheimer's Disease' is not one illness but rather a heterogeneous group of conditions that are intimately related to the normal aging process in the brain. Arne developed what he called empirical semantics as a part of his philosophy. He would have loved to debate the misuse of words like 'Alzheimer's' and 'dementia' in the world and urged us towards a greater appreciation of the power of words and stories, rather than molecules and drugs. Thank you, Arne, for your life, your inspiration and your stories.

Note: For those interested, the video 'The Call of the Mountain' is available at www.dailymotion.com/video/x8meah_arne-naess_creation. The film includes interviews of Arne in his hut in the mountains and demonstrates his vigorous lifestyle and manner of thinking.

Chapter 15

Nature, Spiritual Care and Dementia from an Asian Perspective

MANJIT KAUR NIJJAR

This study is based on a Punjabi Community living in the United Kingdom. Anecdotal evidence was collected from three carers looking after someone with dementia over a number of years and two people living with dementia. The third person has advanced dementia so was unable verbally to express their experiences.

The examples are based on their experiences and are as individual as the progression of dementia can be. All the carers were born in the United Kingdom and the people with dementia were born in the Punjab region of either India or Pakistan. All names have been changed to protect their identities.

There were a number of difficulties that arose in the early days around the experiences and expectations of the carers and the person with dementia. The carers' experiences and expectations were defined predominantly by their lives in the UK and the societal conventions they adhered to whilst navigating two distinct cultures. This meant that they found they lacked knowledge of their parents' lives in Northern India or Pakistan. This was compounded by the lack of communication on the part of the older generation, who were reluctant to talk about their lives before arriving in the UK. This in itself presented a barrier to understanding the needs of the person with dementia and their spiritual needs, because the carers had a traditional image of religion being the only route to spirituality. This was reinforced by the religious leaders and by statutory services when asking about the person with dementia's religious beliefs.

The realisation that there was a connection between nature and spiritual awareness (Figure 15.1), whether in the form of the seasons, the moon, the feel of heat and soil or the love of animals came either through reminiscence-based work or through observations made over a period of time.

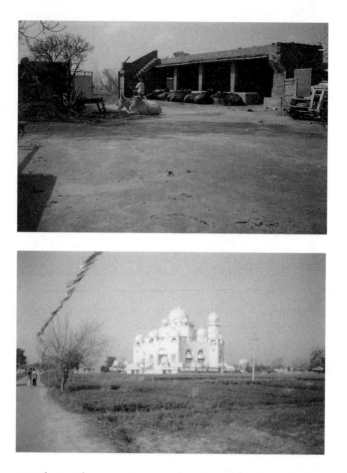

Figure 15.1 The Punjabi community, particularly those born and raised in the Punjab, recognises a connection between nature and spiritual awareness
Photos: S. Herian

For the older generations of the Punjabi community, agriculture has played a large part in their lives. Although the people with dementia in this study came to the UK in the late 1950s and the 1960s, that connection to nature has manifested itself through the continued celebration of festivals and ceremonies. Whilst living in Northern India or Pakistan, these people lived with a greater awareness of nature, as their livelihoods depended upon it. The different seasons defined what activities would take place at these particular times, such as planting and harvesting, etc.

Mrs S

Mrs S followed her husband to the UK in the late 1950s after growing up in Pakistan, but then moved to India. All of her five children were born in England. She was diagnosed with dementia in 1998 and her daughter, Kal, is her sole carer. Kal has kept a journal chronicling her experiences as a carer. As a result of doing this, she has established some patterns in her mother's behaviour coinciding with the change of seasons and the moon.

Kal has noted that, in the nights preceding a full moon, her mother becomes unsettled and is unable to sleep. On the night of the full moon her mother will sit up in bed and mutter about her experiences of living in Pakistan. She will continually repeat the same things, particularly about the village where she lived. Kal feels that the full moon makes her mother regress back to her childhood, to the partition of India and Pakistan, and that she relives those memories. She becomes very anxious and her eyes dart around the room almost as if she is expecting something to happen.

Depending on the interpretation of the lunar calendar the new moon signifies the beginning of a month for some, whilst for others it is the full moon that represents the beginning of a new month.

Within the Punjabi culture, some consider the full moon to be the bearer of mischief or the time to purge malevolent elements from one's life. This may give an indication of the rationale behind the behaviour of Mrs S.

Through keeping a journal, Kal has also noticed that her mother's energy levels are directly linked to seasonal changes. Her mother's sleeping patterns and her desire for activity decrease during the autumn and winter months, and conversely increase during the spring and summer months.

During the spring and summer months Kal's mother is more alert and her eyes are more expressive. She will become more talkative. In the autumn and winter she is less responsive and becomes increasingly introverted.

For Kal, keeping the journal has allowed her to reflect on her mother's moods and behaviours with particular reference to nature. This experiential information has provided her with reassurance, security and confidence in her ability to care for her mother.

Mrs T

Mrs T came from Pakistan to live in the UK with her husband in the late 1960s. Of her eight children, five were born in the UK. She goes to Pakistan every year on a pilgrimage to holy sites in Northern Pakistan with members of her family. She was diagnosed with dementia in 2009. She is cared for by her son, Sajid and his family, but also has a large family support network living nearby.

Going to Pakistan provides a safe and familiar environment where Mrs T is more confident in her surroundings and explores alternative types of therapy, including the environment. Aside from the formal observance of her religious beliefs, Mrs T spends the majority of her days in the open air, even sleeping outside, weather permitting.

She says, 'There is different air in Pakistan, the heat is dry and there is a peace that I find in the air that doesn't exist here. The air here clings to you. In Pakistan it soothes you. It lifts your spirits.'

Many Indians and Pakistani people go to the Indian subcontinent during the winter months as a form of remedy for physical and mental ailments, citing the difference in the air as one of the reasons for doing so.

Within the Punjabi cultures of Northern India and Pakistan, air plays a vital role in spirituality, as it is said to cleanse the soul and heal the body. This also extends to the cleansing of homes and businesses. It expunges stagnant emotions and encourages spiritual and physical growth.

Within a historical agricultural context, the cross-fertilisation of crops and flowers through wind pollination, albeit small, would give the notion of the air as a spiritual form more credence, as it promoted life.

Mrs T has a family home and farm where she lives when in Pakistan. Mrs T frequently walks barefoot, feeling the earth beneath her feet and touching the wheat, which, she has stated reinforces her connection to the earth. She says that the power of the earth can be felt through the soil and the growing plants. She has commented that the heat that is expelled by the soil and wheat when growing has healing properties.

Her family have noted that their mother's behaviour and mood becomes more positive and calmer whilst in Pakistan and feel that she has a sense of purpose, particularly during the winter planting season, as she says she can see the wheat growing in the fields.

Having grown up in an agricultural environment, this connection to the earth is understandable, especially as it would have sustained her family and revives memories of her life before moving to the UK.

The difficulty the family has is maintaining that level of inner peace and calmness when their mother is back in the UK. Her behaviour can become quite volatile and she is very frustrated by the lack of freedom in the UK.

Sajid and his wife have tried various techniques to try to pacify and divert Mrs T. Although it is not a part of their religious practices, Sajid and his wife have found that the burning of incense appears to make Mrs T more settled. It appeals to the senses and reminds her of flowers such as roses and jasmine which can be found in the family home in Pakistan.

Incense is used in Hindu and Sikh formal religious practices as a conduit for spiritual awakening through meditation. Many incense brands are named after flowers.

Mr N

Mr N came to England in the early 1960s, having lived in both India and Pakistan. He married and raised his family in the UK. He was diagnosed with dementia in 2005 and was cared for by his son and daughter.

His children were conscious that the formal approach to spirituality via religion was not benefiting him. He had suffered some discrimination at the local Gurdwara (Sikh Temple) because of his dementia. The congregation had withdrawn from him and he found this very difficult to understand.

By pure coincidence his children discovered their father's love of dogs through watching a film on television. This provided them with opportunities for reminiscence. Mr N's children had been unaware that Mr N had owned dogs in India, so when Mr N began reminiscing about the dogs it opened up new avenues for them to explore. It also meant that his children felt that they knew Mr N, the man, better, as opposed to him just being 'Dad'. Mr N's children were surprised about this aspect of his life, as he had never owned dogs in the UK or shown any interest in them.

Mr N would talk at length about his dogs and their characters. One was timid and would 'shake hands' with people, whilst the other one would drag him around the village just so he could bite someone. Mr N showed a profound love for Moti ('diamond'), the dog who would continually misbehave at every given opportunity.

Mr N would talk about his dogs as if they were human and his children became aware that the interaction with dogs gave Mr N a sense of security. Mr N would comment on the dogs he met and compare them to his dogs in India, particularly Moti.

Mr N's children concluded that the spiritual benefit that he received from the dogs created a sense of joy, security and peace for him, something that formal religion was not able to do. This encouraged Mr N's children to contact their neighbour who had dogs, to allow Mr N to spend time with them. The dogs made him feel valued regardless of his own deteriorating mental and physical health. His children also thought that the dogs provided Mr N with unconditional love, which was not being replicated anywhere else in his life. In turn, the dogs accepted Mr N despite his frailties.

There have been many studies showing the beneficial aspects of animal companions; indeed many residential homes have pets.

Conclusion

Within the different faiths of the carers and the people with dementia there is an underlying principle that spirituality has a much broader context and extends to nature. However, ritualised or orthodox religious practices make it difficult to explore this aspect of spirituality, particularly when the person is living with dementia. This may indicate a lack of understanding of dementia, as opposed to any deliberate attempt to exclude contact with nature as a form of therapy or a means of understanding behaviours exhibited by the person with dementia. Spirituality needs to be seen as being a much more fluid and broader concept than that defined by current understanding.

For Indian and Pakistani people with dementia living in the UK, it means that this aspect of their lives and identity often gets overlooked. Once the carers understood this it became easier for them to understand the needs and some of the behaviours of the person with dementia.

Up and Away
and
An Eyeshot in Summer[1]

JOHN KILLICK

Up and Away

Sometimes you can see where
the smoke blows right across
from the factories. Beautiful trees.
Apple blossom. It's a favourite place of mine –
wouldn't it be of yours?

Well I'll have to be off now –
temporary circumstances.

When it's stormy there
we used to nip over.
All the apples got blown off.
That's where most of them lie,
over the terrace and over the garden.

Well I'll be on my road
or they'll be getting the guns out.

Sometimes I think about running away.
Right up through the meadow
to the cliff. It's reasonably steep.
Always keep myself in trim.
There's no change in this place.

Well I'm still on a tether
so I'll have to be getting back.

---

1   The two poems above are composed from the words of people with dementia, and
published in John Killick (ed.) (2009) *Dementia Diary: Poems and Prose.* London: Hawker.

An Eyeshot in Summer

A little eyesight in the middle,
some of it retained for a purpose.

I can see a sleeve of purple.
And then there is yellow in the sky.

The trees are good and dry,
young and barking.

It's a wonderful setting,
this whole melting scene.

Is it opening or seizing?
The view – it's got the ring of expand.

Concluding Reflections

JANE GILLIARD AND MARY MARSHALL

We very much hope that readers have found inspiration, encouragement and ideas from this book. We are acutely aware of its limitations. We hope to inspire dialogues and conversations. We see this book very much as a first step. There need to be a great many books on this important issue. Indeed, we would go so far as to suggest that there might usefully be books on:

- more practical examples

- design of outside spaces (the Dementia Services Development Centre in Stirling aims to publish a book on the design of outside spaces)   .

- cultural issues, since we know that different cultures have different attitudes to outside space

- animals and birds in dementia care.

It has not been easy to sift out the key themes of this book. One is clearly the difference between nature which is relatively domestic (in the sense of tame or farm animals and gardens and farms) and nature which is relatively wild. We would suggest that people need both, but that either is better than nothing.

Our authors, being enthusiasts, have not emphasised many drawbacks, difficulties or risks. Clearly these exist and need attention and planning. David McNair mentions the dangers of too much sun as well as the importance of some sun. Marcus Fellows and his colleagues chose their animals with care.

Another issue our authors did not emphasise, but which is clearly important, is understanding the cultural background of residents. Some cultures are not at all enthusiastic about dogs in the house or the keeping of pigs, for example. This knowledge of cultural attitudes and beliefs is part of person-centred care and we have assumed this to be in place. However, each individual will also have had different experiences of nature, some good and some bad. It is important to know about this when planning activities linked to nature. Some people are scared of water, for example, having had some traumatic childhood experience. Others have a great deal of expertise and experience in growing vegetables, as is shown in Lorraine Robinson's piece on allotments. One of the Hiking Group struggled on stiles, although this turned out to be a positive challenge for the group.

Another theme might be that owners and managers of care homes may need ideas on how to make the best use of outside spaces, in which case we hope to have provided some good ideas such as the potential for creative use of being outside in Claire Craig's chapter. We have not tried to provide a wholly practical book because we wanted it to be just as much an 'ideas' book – which is why we have input on climate change from Peter Whitehouse and his colleagues and a chapter on spirituality by Malcolm Goldsmith. We do not feel these things are separate. They all connect, as everything in nature does.

We conclude from our authors' contributions that you have to believe in the importance of nature and make the best of what you have got. Thus the building in Murcia (Chapter 12) made a special place out of an unlikely site and at Neville Williams House the steep slope in the garden, which was unusable, was made into an asset (Chapter 8).

It never ceases to surprise us that this book is necessary because it is possible that people in many care homes never go outside. Contact with nature is so much part of every person's identity. Even if we cannot go out, we may open windows and doors to let the fresh air in. Nature touches all our senses. We see the colours of the trees in autumn. We hear the birdsong. We feel the soft moss or the crunchy leaves. We smell the flowers or even, as the grandmother of one of us was wont to say, the fresh air. We taste the raindrop on our lip or the salt in the sea air. We use metaphors about nature all the time when we talk about 'strong as an oak' or a 'sunny temperament'. We are all part of nature and suffer if this connection is not reinforced all the time, or is even severed. We must have contact with nature for our physical, mental and spiritual health. People with dementia in care homes are fellow citizens and we all must ensure that they have the same opportunities as we have, to relate to and be part of nature.

The Editors

Jane Gilliard is a social worker who has worked in dementia care for over 25 years. She established Dementia Voice, the dementia services development centre for Southwest England, and was its director from 1997 to 2005; she chaired the National Network of Dementia Services Development Centres; was a member of the National Institute for Clinical Excellence (NICE)/Social Care Institute for Excellence (SCIE) Guideline Development Group; and sat on the Working Group that developed the National Dementia Strategy for England.

Mary Marshall is a social worker who has worked with and for older people for most of her professional career. She was the director of the Dementia Services Development Centre at the University of Stirling from 1989 until she retired in 2005. She now writes and lectures on dementia care. She chaired the steering group for the new dementia standards in Scotland.

The Contributors

Halldóra Arnardóttir, a member of the architecture office SARQ, is an art historian with a PhD from the Bartlett, University College London. She has written extensively on art, design and architecture around Europe. Now she coordinates the investigation 'Art and Culture as Therapy' on non-pharmacological treatment for Alzheimer's disease at the Hospital Virgen de la Arrixaca in Murcia, Spain.

Simone de Bruin is a researcher at the National Institute for Public Health and the Environment in Bilthoven, the Netherlands. She undertook her PhD research at Wageningen University, the Netherlands, which focused on day care at green care farms for older people with dementia.

Claire Craig is an occupational therapist with a particular interest in the potential of the arts to promote well-being for people with dementia. She currently works at the Art and Design Centre, Sheffield Hallam University where her post spans the areas of occupational therapy and art and design research. She lives in Yorkshire and enjoys nothing more than walking her dog in the countryside, which she considers as being integral to her physical and mental well-being.

Marie-José Enders-Slegers works at the Department of Clinical and Health Psychology of Utrecht University, the Netherlands. She has researched the effects of animal-assisted interventions and 'green care' on vulnerable populations (e.g. people with dementia and people with mental health problems).

Danny George is Assistant Professor in the College of Medicine at the Penn State University, PA, USA. Also an aspiring artist, he is from Cleveland, Ohio and earned his BA in English and Philosophy from the College of Wooster (OH) and his MSc and PhD in Medical Anthropology from Oxford University.

Marcus Fellows has been chief executive of the charity Broadening Choices for Older People (BCOP) for 12 years, having previously worked in the private and the public care sector. He is also involved in both management consultancy and lecturing for charity and academic organisations throughout the world. BCOP runs many services for older people.

Malcolm Goldsmith was ordained in the Church of England in 1962, and worked in parishes in Birmingham, Nottingham and Edinburgh, and as a university chaplain and a chaplain to a hospice. He was a Research Fellow within the Dementia Services Development Centre at the University of Stirling, and wrote and lectured widely on issues related to ageing and dementia, including two books, *In A Strange Land: People with dementia and the local church* (2004, 4M Publications) and *Hearing the Voice of People with Dementia: Opportunities and obstacles* (2002, Jessica Kingsley Publishers).

Brian Hennell was born in London in 1938, and worked for central government as a manager. In 1990 he became a house husband following a severe road crash. As he was an avid reader, the diagnosis of frontal temporal dementia in 2009 impacted greatly, for he had difficulty following plots and themes.

A move to Gloucestershire to live near his sons and their families opened up new horizons and challenges for Brian. Together with June, he has featured in DVDs focusing on living well with dementia, read scripts from autocues like a professional and taken part in training sessions for care home staff. He loves Gloucestershire and his new home beside the Stroudwater Navigation Canal and so does labrador Jack.

June Hennell has always been people-focused in her career, firstly in training and human resources and latterly specialising in conflict resolution and adjudication for the Centre of Excellence in Employment Law. Bringing up three children and hosting more than 500 foreign guests from 41 different countries from 1992 until 2009 prepared June for the flexibility required to adapt to living well with dementia.

Recently June has written and delivered dementia training material, inspired the production of the award-winning *Living Well Handbook* (2010, NHS Gloucestershire), and cooperated with a range of statutory bodies, voluntary organisations and the media to deliver the message that early diagnosis can be key to living well with dementia.

Lynda Hughes is lead occupational therapist and runs Forget Me Not Centre, a service based in Swindon for people diagnosed with early-onset dementia. With a passion to promote positive and inclusive attitudes towards dementia, she supports individuals and groups to accept and adapt to the challenges of dementia, facilitating support, participation and hope through engagement in occupation. She regularly teams up with her clients in a wide variety of public speaking, teaching, and media work to promote acceptance, awareness and inclusion.

Innovations in Dementia is a community interest company (CIC), working in a positive way with people with dementia. Their goal is to see people with dementia remain part of their local communities and their own lives, no matter how advanced their dementia.

Trevor Jarvis is 69 years old and was diagnosed with vascular dementia in 2001 following a severe stroke. He has been happily married to Ann for 43 years and has two sons aged 41 and 38, and three wonderful grandchildren aged five, eight and 13, who are without question the apple of his eye. His dearest passion is his garden – never a Kew but forever his bit of 'England's Greenest Land', and his wife says it has kept him out of trouble for years!

Brett Joseph is an environmental educator and farmer/permaculturalist with a background in humanistic-transpersonal psychology and environmental law. He recently launched the Center for Ecological Culture, Inc., a non-profit organisation dedicated to empowering place-based communities in the areas of environmental health and social justice. While pursuing his PhD in organizational systems at Saybrook University, CA, USA, he currently serves The Intergenerational School and its community as in-house educational researcher, gardener, and legal advisor for kinship clients.

John Killick has worked as a poet with people with dementia for 17 years, currently for Alzheimer Scotland. In 2009 he wrote *The Elephant in the Room* (Cambridgeshire Libraries). His most recent publication is *Creativity and Communication in Persons with Dementia*, co-authored with Claire Craig (2011, Jessica Kingsley Publishers).

Rachael Litherland has worked with older people and people with dementia for the past 13 years. With a background in psychology and advocacy, she developed and managed the national 'Living with Dementia' programme for the Alzheimer's Society between 2000 and May 2006. This included providing leadership on issues relating to the involvement and support of people with dementia and supporting people with dementia in service and information development, campaigning and self-advocacy. She is now a director of Innovations in Dementia, a community interest company that works on positive projects with people with dementia.

Neil Mapes is the founder and director of Dementia Adventure, a social enterprise venture created to take people with dementia out into nature. He is also a Clore Social Fellow, a Visiting Fellow at the University of Essex and an UnLtd Awardee. Neil can often be found tending his allotment or running around the Essex countryside.

James McKillop is married with four children. He led an ordinary sort of life and his life was his family. The family had a rough time before diagnosis, as his behaviour had changed. Luckily with treatment and support they are now back to a family unit.

With the support he gets from his family, his medication and dedicated support workers, James now plays an active part in the community and is on many committees, some unconnected with dementia but related, for example, to learning difficulties. He gives many talks to encourage others with the illness and carers, to make the best of their lives.

David McNair has been a lighting engineer since 1975 and is a Fellow of the Institution of Lighting Professionals. He was president of the Institution in 2003 and has presented papers at many lighting conferences. Presently he is an independent lighting specialist, working with the Dementia Services Development Centre, University of Stirling, Scotland, to acquire and disseminate knowledge on the benefits of good lighting for people with dementia.

Manjit Kaur Nijjar is a former carer for her father. She currently works in Wolverhampton with families living with dementia.

Simon Oosting is assistant professor at the Department of Animal Sciences at Wageningen University, the Netherlands. His specialisation is the role and functions of animals and farming systems with animals in societies.

The Park Club (Age Concern, Exeter) is a day centre specialising in supporting older people with memory problems. Individuals have the opportunity to get involved with different things and tap into things that they enjoy. They are always keen to influence the wider world.

Ann Rainsford is the manager of Neville Williams House. She has been employed by BCOP for the last 32 years and has held many posts in her time with the company. Her passion has always been to work and care for elderly people. She started her career as a hairdresser, and after having her third child decided to go into semi-retirement – but not for long! She was offered part-time work at a BCOP nursing home that was on her doorstep and she could not refuse the chance to give care and support to the people who had given so much to the country we live in. She started her new venture as a care assistant, and after many years of hard work raising a family and achieving care qualifications, now very proudly holds the position of Registered Manager at Neville Williams House, which she is enjoying immensely.

Lorraine Robertson is the services manager at West Dunbartonshire Services, Alzheimer Scotland. She has worked with a variety of client groups, in different sectors for 33 years and has been with Alzheimer Scotland since 2008.

Javier Sánchez Merina, an architect, is the director of the architecture office SARQ, lecturer of design at Alicante University (Spain) and Alzheimer's disease researcher included in the list of supporters of the global Campaign to Prevent Alzheimer's Disease by 2020 (PAD2020).

Jos Schols holds a chair in Elderly Care Medicine at Maastricht University, the Netherlands. His research focuses on care innovations for frail and disabled older people, and specifically on improving medical care for this target group.

The Scottish Dementia Working Group is the independent voice of people with dementia within Alzheimer Scotland. It is a campaigning and awareness-raising group whose members all have a diagnosis of dementia.

Peter Whitehouse is a geriatric neurologist, cognitive neuroscientist and environmental bioethicist at Case Western Reserve University and University Hospitals Case Medical Center in Cleveland, Ohio, USA. He co-founded The Intergenerational School (www.tisonline.org) with his wife, Cathy, and serves as Director of Adult Education, where his interests include multimedia narrative and sustainable learning organisations. He is the author of many articles and several books, including *The Myth of Alzheimer's: What You Aren't Being Told about Today's Most Dreaded Diagnosis* (2008, St Martin Press).

Johanna Wigg is a social gerontologist committed to advancing the field of dementia research at The Vicarage by the Sea, ME, USA. She engages in daily, direct care of elders living with dementing illnesses, while simultaneously conducting research that seeks to increase knowledge concerning the social care of individuals living with dementia. Johanna is an independent consultant on dementia care who lectures, teaches, and is currently writing about alternative approaches to long-term dementia care.

Subject Index

Author Index